P9-DUN-022

Contents

Most children have plenty of energy, but that doesn't mean they're fit. You—the parent—can make a difference.

Being able to make fast tracks from the couch to the refrigerator doesn't mean your child's in good shape. Learn how your child measures up on four fitness components.

Here are practical and proven steps you can take to select goals and activities that match your child's developmental level.

Kids eat more than 30% of their calories in snacks. In addition to 29 healthy snack ideas, you'll learn how to feed a young athlete and how to talk veggies to a two-year-old.

Olympic gymnast Mary Lou Retton remembers how activity "was always a way of life" with her family. This chapter explains how to balance a busy schedule and be a positive influence on your child's fitness.

Innovative and effective physical education programs do exist! With these tips you can recognize and lobby for school programs to improve your child's fitness.

Foreword

You won't believe how wonderful a gift you will be giving your children if you help them to develop an active lifestyle and good eating habits. As a doctor, I can find no elixir or treatment that improves the quality of life better than a healthy lifestyle. It seems so simple that many people can't believe it's true.

Over the years we doctors have prescribed a variety of treatments to fight disease. But the best prescription I can give anyone to reduce the risk of heart disease, obesity, diabetes, and many cancers is to encourage an active lifestyle and a lowfat diet. This is true for you and your kids.

Of course, it's easy for me as a doctor to say fit kids are healthier kids. Being a parent and helping your child learn about the joys of active living is a different story, you protest. But, you see, I'm not only a doctor, I'm a parent too. Actually, I'm a grandparent now. And I know you alone can't do everything for your children. You must reach out to your medical community, to your child's school and teachers, and to the community. And that's where Your Child's Fitness comes in.

By reading *Your Child's Fitness* you will be taking the first of many steps to help your child develop an active lifestyle. Active living is an ongoing process. What sport your child enjoys at age 9 may change by junior high school and again by high school. This book will help you not only to help your child select age-appropriate activities but also to develop patterns and attitudes in your child that will last well into adulthood. And that is the secret of a successful youth fitness program—empowering your child with knowledge and abilities he or she can and will use to make healthy choices.

And choices there are! There is no one perfect sport, just as there is no one perfect treatment or medicine. What sports are good for your child? What options do you have regarding youth programs? How do you select healthy foods? You will find answers to these questions and more in *Your Child's Fitness*.

I've been physically active for more than 60 years—most of my life. But there has not been one sport or one diet that I've followed. My choices have changed as my family developed. When I didn't have kids, I set *personal* fitness goals. Once I had children, my fitness goals included their needs as well. And now that they are grown, I have a new set of goals. What has remained constant is my wholehearted love of physical activity—the fulfillment of reaching a goal, the sense of accomplishment in mastering a new sport. I learned these wonderful feelings from my parents, and I tried to pass them on to our children. Give your children the tools they can use to develop, master, and adapt their fitness programs to their stage in life.

So read on! I think you will enjoy Susan's breezy style and thoughtful outlook. She's been promoting physical fitness—expounding the truths, expelling the myths—for almost 15 years. And as a parent, she can relate to your busy schedule, as well as to the lofty dreams you may have for your children. Remember, there is no better gift than empowering your child with an active lifestyle.

Ronald M. Lawrence, PhD, MD
Founder
American Medical Athletic Association
American Academy of Sports Physicians

Acknowledgments

I have always enjoyed team sports and *Your Child's Fitness* is truly a team effort. First and foremost, I would like to thank Rainer Martens for asking me to write *Your Child's Fitness*. Rainer's vision and hard work have made an incredible impact on the health and fitness of America's children. And since he knows more about kid's fitness than I will ever know, it was an incredible honor to write this book for him. I would also like to thank all of the other wonderful people I've met through Human Kinetics, especially Ted Miller, for their good ideas and guidance.

I have been extremely lucky to have worked for more than 14 years with the American Running and Fitness Association, a nonprofit association of recreational athletes and sports medicine professionals who come together to educate and motivate people about developing and maintaining a regular exercise program. AR&FA has an abundance of very talented advisors who volunteer their time to be sure that we provide accurate, useful information to the public. Without the resources of AR&FA this book could not have been written.

Youth fitness is an evolving science. I know that the physical fitness of America's children will improve in the coming years because many talented individuals are focusing on this issue. I am extremely grateful for the inspiration and ideas I have received from the following fitness leaders: Ken Cooper, MD, Chuck Corbin, PhD, Charles Kuntzleman, EdD, Russ Pate, PhD, Jim Sallis, PhD, Vern Seefeldt, PhD, Charles Sterling, EdD, Wynn Updyke, PhD, and Judy Young, PhD. Their thoughts and ideas permeate *Your Child's Fitness*.

I would also like to thank all the talented people who put up with me on a day-to-day basis. My current friends at AR&FA, Lorie Allion and Barbara Baldwin, and my old friends there, Julie Wisor, Lisa Gundling, and Scott Douglas, all helped me find time to get this project off the ground and gave me guidance along the way. A special thanks also goes to Nancy Best, who has more chutzpah than you can imagine and who opened many doors to get all of the sports celebrities involved with this project. I would also like to thank Doug Brown for providing most of the photographs for the book. And to think I thought his expertise was on the croquet course!

And last, I need to say a very special thanks to those on my home front. Both Virginia Zambrana and Nguyet Le Vu, two fabulous parents, who helped keep my family safe and happy so that I had the confidence to spend the extra time on this project. Thanks also go to my parents who gave me tremendous support, both verbally and in baby-sitting, because, well, that's the kind of parents they have always been. And my loving and adorable husband John deserves extra kisses and thanks for his support and encouragement. He put his painting on hold for two years so I could have the space to work on my creativity. Now it's his turn at bat.

I feel very lucky to be associated with so many team players!

Credits

Table 3.1 is adapted from *Kid Fitness*, by Kenneth H. Cooper, MD, MPH. Copyright © 1991 by Kenneth H. Cooper. Information originally compiled by Dr. Vern Seefeldt.

Table 4.1 is from *Kid Fitness*, by Kenneth H. Cooper, MD, MPH. Copyright © 1991 by Kenneth H. Cooper. Used by permission of Bantam Books, a division of Bantam Doubleday Dell Publishing Group, Inc.

Table 4.2 is from *Kid Fitness*, by Kenneth H. Cooper, MD, MPH. Copyright © 1991 by Kenneth H. Cooper. Used by permission of Bantam Books, a division of Bantam Doubleday Dell Publishing Group, Inc.

Figure 5.1 is adapted from Home and Community in Children's Exercise Habits (The National Children and Youth Fitness Study II). Ross, J., Pate, R., Caspersen, C., Damberg, C., & Svilar, M. (1987). *Journal of Physical Education, Recreation and Dance*, **58**(9), pp. 85–92.

Table 5.2 is from *American Youth and Sports Participation*, a study sponsored by the Athletic Footwear Association. Reprinted with permission.

Table 5.3 is from *American Youth and Sports Participation*, a study sponsored by the Athletic Footwear Association. Reprinted with permission.

Table 8.2 is reproduced by permission of *Pediatrics* vol. 81, page 737, copyright 1988.

Table 9.1 is from *Kid Fitness*, by Kenneth H. Cooper, MD, MPH. Copyright © 1991 by Kenneth H. Cooper. Used by permission of Bantam Books, a division of Bantam Doubleday Dell Publishing Group, Inc.

The testing sections in chapter 2 (page 17 "Who Should Conduct the Test?" through the first paragraph on page 30) are from the Prudential FITNESSGRAM. Reprinted with permission from The Cooper Institute for Aerobics Research, Dallas, Texas.

The poem on page 87 is from *Teaching Elementary Physical Education*, **1**(4), January 1, 1993, p. 11. Reprinted with permission from Human Kinetics Publishers.

The quiz, "Does Your School Make the Grade?" on page 102 is from "The Healthy School Quiz," by Charles Kuntzleman, EdD, 1991, *Running & FitNews*, **9**(9). Reprinted with permission.

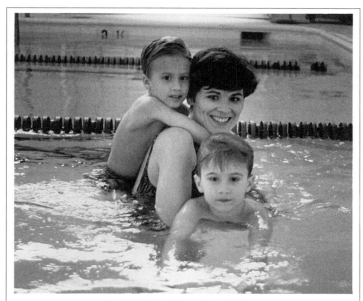

© Doug Brown

1

Children's Fitness: A Challenge for Parents

You'd think growing up was an Olympic sport. Nonstop continuous motion—between school, play groups, scouting, religious activities, music lessons, and the youth league, children and their parents are always on the go. With all this activity our families must be superfit, right?

Wrong. Appearances can be misleading when it comes to fitness. A child who is of average weight and appears healthy may actually have little endurance or strength to carry out daily tasks. A short jog to the bus stop may leave him huffing for minutes. On the other hand, children who are a bit overweight might be much more fit—that is, they may be stronger and more active, not tire as easily, and be more flexible. Despite the extra weight, these kids might make it to the bus stop without breaking a sweat. The goal of this book is to help you direct your energy, and your child's, into something positive—and lasting. It aims at giving you not just good information, but also *useful* and *effective* ideas. And you'll find them in *Your Child's Fitness*.

We all need fitness to meet the demands of living today and into the 21st century. Living isn't merely existing. Our lives, whether we're children or adults, offer a whirlwind of activities, thoughts, relationships, interactions,

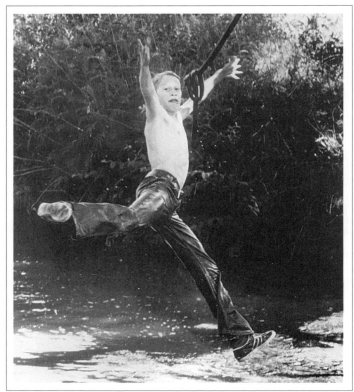

© Doug Brown

and opportunities for pleasure and productivity that require a minimal level of vitality and endurance. Fitness is having the energy to live out our days as we want to.

Fitness is a blessing that you probably wish for your entire family. You can give your child the foundations for lifelong fitness, but this gift is not automatically preserved. What this book will show you is how the family can work together in pursuit of fitness for each member. As parents we can provide a lifestyle that will help our children now and teach them how to live in the future. At the same time, we parents will be improving the quality and fitness of our own lives. You will also read in *Your Child's Fitness* how to tap into resources beyond the home to help give your child greater fitness. You can harness the resources of schools, community organizations, and the medical profession to effectively teach your child about becoming fitter and healthier while having fun in the process.

How Kids Play Today

Your kids may have energy, but if they are more apt to plop in front of the TV with a bag of chips than to be out riding a bike or playing ball with friends, then they may not be as active as you think.

Today's kids find it more difficult to be fit than did their counterparts a generation ago: Television's pull on kids is sophisticated, and video games can gobble up enormous amounts of time (and money!). Parents on average have less time available to spend being active with children. As a child I walked to school, but I don't feel safe letting my kids do that—it's either a bus or a carpool for them. Even children who play sports seldom get enough exercise from the activity, often waiting for a turn or watching teammates. The result? Kids today are less active, less fit. Consider these facts:

- Two of every five children between ages 5 and 8 are obese, have elevated blood pressure and cholesterol, and aren't active.
- Half of all children don't get enough exercise to strengthen the heart and lungs.
- Kids under 10 spend twice the time watching television that they do actively playing. There is a direct relationship between TV time and body fatness—the more they watch the tube, the more likely they are to have excess body fat.

The sad truth is, kids today are more sedentary, weigh more, and have more body fat than children did 20 years ago. Only one of three kids from ages 6 to 17 meets the minimum standards for cardiovascular fitness, flexibility, and abdominal and upper body strength. How will these kids

Did You Know?

By 7th grade children's participation in sports and fitness begins to drop and never rises again. Many children give up because they believe they aren't as athletically inclined as their peers.

function as adults? The American College of Sports Medicine recommends that children spend at least 20 minutes three days a week participating in vigorous physical activity. In the 1984 National Children and Youth Fitness Study, 62% of the students in grades 10 through 12 reported doing this much activity or more. Yet by 1994, that "active student" figure had dropped to 37%.

The news on children's fitness isn't all bad. A 1990 study of kids between the ages of 6 and 17 done by Wynn Updyke at Indiana University showed gains between 1980 and 1989 for boys and girls in strength and endurance of abdominal and hip flexor muscles (assessed by sit-ups). Boys regained arm and shoulder strength, and girls improved in upper body strength. Improvements were also shown in flexibility of the back and hamstrings (muscles in the back of the thigh).

But according to Updyke's Chrysler/AAU research, even this good news was offset by declines in stamina. And the improvements in strength are still short of what could reasonably be expected. Many girls were unable to hold up their body weight in a flexed-arm hang. Sadder still, girls begin to show measurable declines in strength and endurance by age 14—hardly an inevitable situation when, in fact, women age 85 and older are capable of still building strength and increasing endurance.

Poor fitness levels don't just result in poor sports performance. Today's real issue is that poor fitness produces children with low self-esteem, poor body images, and not enough energy to be at their best. What's worse, they are more likely to grow up to be sedentary adults with these same traits and are more likely to develop cancer and heart disease in adulthood.

Shaking Up Sedentary Parents

Children need to develop healthy behaviors, and parents are in the best position to teach them. We parents hold an enormous power over our children, and we have an active role to play. But all the advice in the world to your child about fitness won't mean much if your own approach to fitness is poor.

> **M**y family has always motivated me to be active. My dad was always active playing professional baseball. And my mom was active too. They always encouraged us to be active and to try a variety of sports
>
> Cal Ripken, Jr.
> *professional baseball player*
> *(Baltimore Orioles)*

A parent's attitude and activity level have an enormous impact on a child. If you're active, chances are your child is too. But if the only time you break into a jog is to get a snack between TV commercials, then your child may not care much about exercise either. If you smoke or drink in excess, graze on junk food, or burn the candle at both ends, you're sending unhealthy messages to your child. It's not good enough to tell your son—as you puff on a cigarette in your easy chair—that he shouldn't smoke. Your smoker's cough speaks louder than your words!

Take a moment to consider how you influence your child regarding fitness. Are you inactive? Do you use TV to occupy your child rather than encouraging her to play outside? Are you "too busy" to make time for activity with your child? Would you sooner zap a hot dog in the microwave than clean a raw vegetable? If you answered *yes* to any of those questions, you should consider changing your behaviors for the sake of both you and your child.

Did You Know?

Most symptoms of aging are due to atrophy—the "use it or lose it" phenomenon. As people age they often choose to not be so active. Then when they do exercise, they tire easily and become sore. Age isn't the culprit—a sedentary lifestyle is!

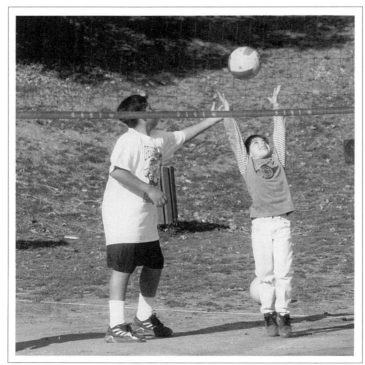

© Doug Brown

Left to their own devices, children are innately active. We are born with a love of movement and feel better when we are strong and vigorous. The same goes for a healthy diet. Toddlers rarely overeat—they can naturally regulate how much food and drink they need. And children naturally enjoy a variety of vegetables and fruits. So where do they pick up so many unhealthy habits?

You guessed it. We have seen the enemy, and the enemy is us! It's easier to keep watch over children watching TV than playing outdoors. It's easier to keep children at home than to take them to a community recreation center to play ball. It's easier to hand children a bag of chips than to make a sandwich. And so we take the easy way out—at our children's expense.

Children are a reflection of their parents, and their society. If children are taught by sedentary, overweight teachers, brought up by inactive parents, and watch their grandparents retire only to sink into armchairs, it should surprise nobody that youngsters follow the examples they see. Most parents are not fit. Half of the parents with children in grades 1 to 4 never exercise. Less than a third exercise the basic amount needed for good health.

Our children are on the fast track to an unnecessarily early grave. Don't use the excuse that you weren't athletic when you were young and you turned out okay. It is very unlikely that as a child you watched as much television, drank as much soda, had as little physical education at school, and played as many video games as your child does. Things are different today. It's almost as if there is a concentrated effort to tranquilize children instead of invigorate them.

It's up to us to turn this problem around. The good news is that we can do it if we work together. Researchers, physical educators, coaches, recreation directors, fitness instructors, and parents like you and me can make a difference. The schools can teach a curriculum for lifetime activities—sports you can play at any age—and our community programs are expanding past competitive team leagues.

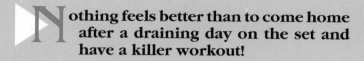

Nothing feels better than to come home after a draining day on the set and have a killer workout!

Mario Lopez
teen actor
("Saved by the Bell")

Awakening Sedentary Kids

So how do you help your child become more fit? Fitness is a way of life. It's not confined to what your child does in physical education class or on the tennis court in the summer. It's not something gained solely through exercise or good diet or by abstaining from unhealthy behaviors, like smoking. Fitness comes from consistently making healthy choices: getting regular exercise, eating well, getting proper sleep, and choosing activities that increase flexibility, coordination, endurance, and strength.

This book will help you understand a variety of practical ways you can help your child be more fit. We'll explore children's fitness from various perspectives: the schools, community programs, the medical community. I'll help you assess your child's diet. And we'll examine ways you can help your child stay on a healthy track throughout life.

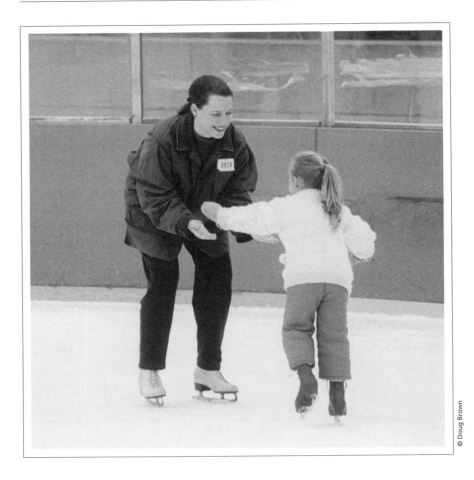

© Doug Brown

Being Fit Together

Regular, gentle activity—we're not talking triathlons here, just walking, yard work, swimming—can reduce the risk of developing heart disease, diabetes, and many forms of cancer. Eating a lowfat diet is another way to avoid these same diseases and obesity. Exercise makes you stronger, more productive, and often better coordinated. Physical health through an active lifestyle is also associated with a positive self-image, confidence, a feeling of control, and a reduced risk of depression. And given that more than a fourth of all adolescents say they have considered suicide, the benefits of physical activity on mental health are important to consider.

You can combat unhealthy messages, attitudes, and behaviors and positively influence your child's fitness. Just commit yourself to doing these three things to emphasize health and fitness in your family and you'll see quick results:

1. Send positive verbal and nonverbal messages about fitness to your child, and counteract the messages your child may be receiving from other sources that say fitness isn't important.

2. Be fit and healthy yourself! Being a healthy role model is very important; I'll discuss this more in chapter 3.

3. Take a vigorous interest in your child's fitness. Exercise with your child and foster an appreciation for an active, healthy lifestyle.

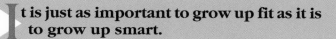

It is just as important to grow up fit as it is to grow up smart.

Arnold Schwarzenegger
actor and fitness advocate

Yes, there are many reasons to be concerned about your child's fitness. But fortunately there are even more ways you can help your child be more fit. It will help if you understand the components of fitness and can gauge just how fit your child is. Parents are the single most influential factor regarding how active and healthy our children will be. By reading this book, you are taking a positive step toward making sure your child enjoys a long, healthy, and active life. Take notes. Set goals. Make a difference—today! Move on to chapter 2 (see, I got you moving already!) for information and guidelines.

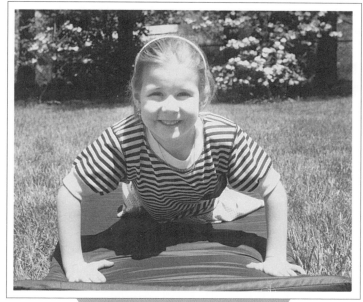

2

Testing Children's Fitness

Fitness comes from consistently making healthy choices about what you do (and don't do) and what you eat. Being fit means, in part, having the physical energy to complete daily activities with ease and pleasure. But if appearances can be deceiving, just how can you determine your child's fitness?

What Fitness Is All About

Let's start with what fitness is *not*. The four components of fitness do not include

- the endurance needed to watch every college bowl game from beginning to end on New Year's day;
- the abdominal strength to push your stomach to its limits on Thanksgiving;
- the balance and agility to carry two sodas in one hand so you can use the other to carry a bag of chips; or
- the coordination required to shove a forkful of food in your mouth while operating the TV remote.

Instead, another four components are more commonly measured to determine fitness: endurance, strength, flexibility, and body composition. Later in the chapter I present a fitness test, the Prudential FITNESSGRAM assessment, for your child that was designed by the Cooper Institute for Aerobics Research. Having these fitness components measured reveals strengths and weaknesses, information you can use to target specific areas to help your child improve.

While scoring high on these four fitness components would be nice, we need to remember that balance and moderation are keys to long-term fitness. Your child needn't become a fitness freak to be healthy.

So before we get down to the sweat of the matter, let's look at how endurance, strength, flexibility, and body composition affect your child's fitness and at ways you can help your child prepare for the test.

Endurance

Endurance is the ability to move or stay active over an extended period. There are two kinds of endurance. *Cardiovascular endurance* means your heart and lungs are strong enough to supply your muscles with fuel over a long haul. Aerobic exercise like walking and swimming that continuously moves major muscle groups such as those in your arms and legs, builds cardiovascular endurance. *Muscular endurance* is the strength to move against resistance for long periods, such as during a long bicycle ride. Lifting weights and climbing stairs build muscle endurance.

We all benefit from improved endurance. Aerobic exercise is the type with the greatest impact on health and disease. With endurance, you can focus your exercise efforts on improving your skills, form, and game strategies because you have the energy to keep on going and going and going—just like the Energizer bunny.

Strength

Strength is the ability to exert a force, whether kicking a ball, lifting a weight, or moving the legs quickly while sprinting. You build strength by working a muscle against resistance. Resistance can be a weight you lift or a hill you climb.

Strength allows you and your child to take on everyday tasks (like mowing the lawn or carrying a heavy backpack home from school) with greater ease. Strength also allows a child to excel in sports by running faster, jumping higher, or throwing farther. A strong back, shoulders, and abdomen are needed to maintain a good posture. And strengthening exercises keep your metabolism up, even after the workout is over, which helps you maintain a healthy body composition. Most important, the risk of getting injured—at home or on the playing field—is less if muscles are strong.

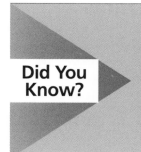

Did You Know?

You can increase your strength while reading this book. Just by contracting a muscle and holding it, you build strength. It's called isometric exercise. As you sit reading, tighten your stomach muscles. Hold them for 30 seconds, then relax. Do this regularly and your clothes will begin to fit more loosely.

Flexibility

How far you can bend your joints depends on your flexibility. Flexibility helps adults and children move more easily and comfortably. And form and posture improve as well, whether on the playing field or sitting at a desk.

The more you stretch, the more flexible you are. Stretching is also relaxing and helps reduce stress and tension. Plus, many fitness professionals believe stretching reduces the risk of developing an injury while playing sports.

Younger people are generally more flexible than older people, so your child probably has no problem here—not! Kids can be as stiff as their parents. Actually, flexibility depends a bit on heredity, a bit on how active you are, and a lot on how much you practice it. Kids who climb trees, do gymnastics, and practice martial arts usually are flexible, but that's because they stretch their muscles and ligaments doing these activities. Most kids who aren't all that fit also aren't all that flexible.

Body Composition

Many Americans put a great emphasis on their body weight, when in fact body composition is more important for determining health and good looks. You want a healthy balance in your body composition between muscle and fat. Because muscles weigh more than fat, the scale is not a reliable measure of body composition.

Many studies are finding that people with too much body fat, as well as people who eat too much fat, have an increased risk of many diseases, including cancer, heart disease, and diabetes. If we help our children maintain a healthy weight at an early age, they are less likely to have weight problems later on. They will also have better self-concepts and will do better at sports and in friendships.

How Active Is Your Child?

Here's a quick quiz that can help you get a handle on how active your child is. Activity and fitness go hand in hand. The more active children are, the more likely they are to be fit (and stay fit). Answer each question and add up your child's score at the end.

How Active Is Your Child?

Quiz

Respond to each question as best you can. Each answer has a numerical value (see the end of the quiz). The higher the number, the better. Add up your responses for a total at the end of the quiz.

1. Does your child have regular instruction in physical education at school?
   a. yes   b. no

2. How many minutes of physical education does your child get each week?
   a. 0   b. 1–60   c. 61–90   d. 90+

3. What percentage of time does your child spend in vigorous activity (i.e., active enough to be short of breath) in physical education?

    a. less than 10% b. 10% to 30% c. 30% to 60% d. more than 60%

4. How many minutes a week does your child have *active* recess?

    a. 0   b. 1–60   c. 61–90   d. 90+

5. Does your child's school administer fitness tests?

    a. yes   b. no

6. Does your child participate in a community-based fitness activity (one organized by the parks and recreation department, a YMCA or YWCA, 4-H, etc.)?

    a. yes   b. no

7. How many of these activities does your child participate in?

Aerobic dance	Archery	Badminton
Baseball	Basketball	Bicycling
Calisthenics	Crew/rowing	Diving
Fencing	Field hockey	Football
Golf	Gymnastics	Hiking/backpacking
Horseback riding	Ice hockey	Jumping rope
Lacrosse	Martial arts	Rodeo
Running	Skating	Skiing
Soccer	Softball	Squash/handball
Swimming	Table tennis	Tennis
Track and field	Volleyball	Walking
Weight lifting	Wrestling	

    a. 0   b. 1 or 2   c. 3 or 4   d. more than 4

8. About how many times a week does your child participate in fitness or sports activities? (All activity counts: school, community, playground, supervised, unsupervised.)

    a. 0   b. 1–3   c. 4–7   d. more than 7

9. Is your child's mother active?

    a. yes   b. no   c. Child doesn't regularly see her.

10. Is your child's dad active?

    a. yes   b. no   c. Child doesn't regularly see him.

11. Do mom and child exercise together?

    a. yes   b. no

12. Do dad and child exercise together?

    a. yes   b. no

13. Is your child's physical education teacher active and supportive of an active lifestyle?

    a. yes   b. no   c. Child doesn't have physical education.
    d. don't know

14. How many hours a day does your child watch TV?

    a. less than 1   b. 1–2   c. 2–3   d. more than 3

15. Do you think your child is fit?

    a. yes   b. no

16. Does your child think she or he is fit?

    a. yes   b. no

✓Scoring

1. a. 10   b. 0
2. a. 0   b. 3   c. 6   d. 9
3. a. 0   b. 6   c. 9   d. 12
4. a. 0   b. 3   c. 9   d. 12
5. a. 5   b. 0
6. a. 10   b. 0
7. a. 0   b. 3   c. 6   d. 9
8. a. 0   b. 6   c. 9   d. 12
9. a. 20   b. 0   c. 5
10. a. 20   b. 0   c. 5
11. a. 20   b. 0
12. a. 20   b. 0
13. a. 10   b. 0   c. 0
14. a. 0   b. –10   c. –20   d. –40
15. a. 5   b. 0
16. a. 10   b. 0

✓Results

More than 99—Great job! Your child is active regularly and has made physical activity a part of her life. Be sure your child is having fun and doing sports because she wants to. Make sure your child's life is balanced.

61 to 99—Good job—your child is active enough to be healthy. Be sure he is enjoying himself and improving his abilities.

21 to 60—Your child is moderately active but probably hasn't established enough lifestyle patterns to make fitness a part of her life. Get her moving!

Under 20—Your child is in trouble. He's not active enough, and many of the factors that will help him get active aren't in place. Read this book carefully and work with your child. His health is in danger.

Fitness Testing 101

Now let's see how fit your child is. Fitness testing has several benefits. It reinforces the importance of fitness, and it points out your child's strengths and weaknesses. It shows how your child is doing compared to fitness standards, and through testing you can chart progression year by year. Children who can see their improvement are often motivated to improve even more or to make similar gains in other areas.

I recommend your child be tested annually. But it might be fun—and encouraging—to test your child both before and after a single season to measure improvement. If this sounds fun, do it—but don't overdo it. Testing of any sort is not a child's favorite thing!

Who Should Conduct the Test?

A trained fitness professional is best qualified to administer fitness tests. Physical educators and exercise specialists are often trained to give them. Check with your child's physical education teacher to see if tests are conducted at school. If not, ask if the teacher can do one. Local health clubs, recreation centers, and sports medicine facilities are other possibilities, though many are accustomed only to testing adults. (If nothing else, you can probably get one of these places to do the body composition testing. Many clubs do it for free for members.)

If you can't find someone who's trained to test your child, then you can administer the following test yourself. But do your best to find someone else to test your child. Think about it—would you have wanted your parents to test you? Personally, it was hard enough for me to show my folks my report cards.

Make Fitness a Team Effort

As I've said before (and will say again throughout the book) you and your child have to have fun with fitness to make it work. And that includes this testing part. Don't get too focused on the numbers. Fitness testing will only give you a ballpark idea of your child's strengths and weaknesses. In many cases, a child's activity level is a better indicator of fitness level than performance on various tests.

Remember that Golden Rule you're always drumming into your child? ("Do unto others . . . ?") Well, what about now? Make fitness testing a partnership. You could probably learn from it. I know it was a humbling experience for me, a lifelong jock who thought she was pretty hot until she got to the upper body stuff. Why not go through all the tests with your child and record your progress, too.

A final note before you test: Help your child prepare by doing some of the exercises together. Within each portion of the test I'll give you samples of how to practice. For a more detailed description of the exercises used for the test, see chapter 3.

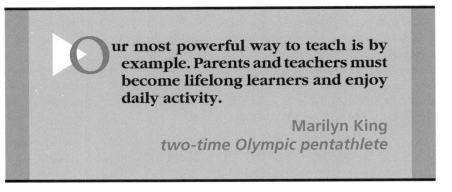

Our most powerful way to teach is by example. Parents and teachers must become lifelong learners and enjoy daily activity.

Marilyn King
two-time Olympic pentathlete

Testing Endurance: The 1-Mile Walk or Run

To measure endurance, have your child walk or run a mile. Time the mile if your child is 10 or older; however, I don't recommend timing children under 10. Their goal should be just to complete a mile. Few, if any, 8- and 9-year-olds think running a mile as fast as they can is fun. And the fun factor is key in most fitness activities.

Getting Ready

Take walks or jog with your child for a month or two before the test. It usually takes 4 to 6 weeks for a person to build up endurance. Take this test on a pleasant day. When it's too hot or too cold, your child won't perform up to par. Hot temperatures and vigorous activity don't go together well.

What You Need

Use a stopwatch or watch with a second hand if you are timing. It's easiest to determine a mile by using an outdoor track. (For most school tracks, there are four laps to a mile. If the track is metric, add 10 yards to the final lap. Talk to a school coach or physical education instructor to find out the distance per lap.)

Doing the Test

Provide support by running with your child or inviting a peer to run, too.

Before beginning, jog or walk easily with your child to warm up. Then as she stands behind the starting mark, say, "Ready, set, go!" and begin timing as soon as she starts moving. Encourage her to start out easily, running or walking at a constant pace. If by the last lap she still feels good, have her increase speed. It is better to start out slowly and speed up at the end than to start too fast and fade out. Don't let your child sit once she's finished the test. Have her walk around for a couple of minutes until her heart and breathing slow down. See Table 2.1 for scoring guidelines.

Table 2.1 1-Mile Run Standards for Endurance					
Boys			**Girls**		
Age	Fit	Needs to improve	Age	Fit	Needs to improve
5	Can	Cannot	5	Can	Cannot
6	complete	complete	6	complete	complete
7	mile by	mile by	7	mile by	mile by
8	walking or	walking or	8	walking or	walking or
9	running	running	9	running	running
10	9:00–11:30*	>11:30	10	9:30–12:30	>12:30
11	8:30–11:00	>11:00	11	9:00–12:00	>12:00
12	8:00–10:30	>10:30	12	9:00–12:00	>12:00
13	7:30–10:00	>10:00	13	9:00–11:30	>11:30
14	7:00–9:30	>9:30	14	8:30–11:00	>11:00
15	7:00–9:00	>9:00	15	8:00–10:30	>10:30
16	7:00–8:30	>8:30	16	8:00–10:00	>10:00
17	7:00–8:30	>8:30	17	8:00–10:00	>10:00
17+	7:00–8:30	>8:30	17+	8:00–10:00	>10:00

*Time given in minutes (i.e., 9:00–11:30 means 9 min to 11 min 30 sec).

Testing Strength: Abdomen

Most fitness tests measure the strength of abdominal muscles because they are very important for posture and healthy backs. The abdominals are also easy to test with an exercise called a curl-up.

Getting Ready

A curl-up is similar to a bent-knee sit-up, but it focuses primarily on stomach muscles and is gentler to the spine than a sit-up. Practice by doing curl-ups, bent-knee sit-ups, and crunches (see p. 41).

To do a curl-up, lie on your back, legs slightly apart, knees slightly bent (about 140 degrees), and feet flat on the floor. Your arms should be straight by your side with palms resting on the floor or mat. With heels touching the ground, curl forward slowly, sliding your fingers toward your feet; then curl back down to your starting position. It often takes one minute to do about 20 curl-ups. No rest is permitted. When your child stops moving, the test is over.

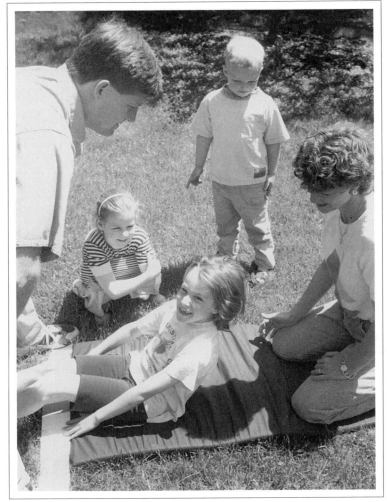

© Doug Brown

What You Need

Perform curl-ups on a carpet or padded mat. A bed or bouncy surface makes the test too easy, and a wooden floor is uncomfortable. You will need a measuring strip (made out of cardboard or paper) to determine how far down the fingers should slide during the curl-up. For children under 10, the strip should be about 30 inches long and 3 inches wide. For children 10 and older, the strip should be 4-1/2 inches wide.

Doing the Test

Once your child is comfortably in place, place the measuring strip under his legs on the mat so that his fingertips are just resting on the edge. A complete curl-up is counted when your child curls up so his fingers slide 3 to 4-1/2 inches across the strip and then he returns to the starting position (for scoring, see Table 2.2). Count out loud, and encourage him as he goes.

Table 2.2	Curl-up Standards for Strength				
Boys			**Girls**		
Age	Fit	Needs to improve	Age	Fit	Needs to improve
5	2–10	<2	5	2–10	<2
6	2–10	<2	6	2–10	<2
7	4–14	<4	7	4–14	<4
8	6–20	<6	8	6–20	<6
9	9–24	<9	9	9–22	<9
10	12–24	<12	10	12–26	<12
11	15–28	<15	11	15–29	<15
12	18–36	<18	12	18–32	<18
13	21–40	<21	13	18–32	<18
14	24–45	<24	14	18–32	<18
15	24–47	<24	15	18–35	<18
16	24–47	<24	16	18–35	<18
17	24–47	<24	17	18–35	<18
17+	24–47	<24	17+	18–35	<18

Did You Know?

Even if you did 100 curl-ups a day, you could still have "love handles." While curl-ups and sit-ups strengthen abdominal muscles, they aren't a great fat burner—and love handles are mostly excess fat. Bulging bellies are due to weak muscles and too much body fat. Combine a lowfat diet with your sit-ups or curl-ups to reduce your belly.

Testing Strength: Upper Body

We suggest a push-up to test your child's upper body strength instead of the more traditional chin-up or pull-up because most kids can't do chin-ups or pull-ups. Why use a test that most people fail? That said, some will have trouble doing a push-up as well. But push-ups are a great exercise that your children can do the rest of their lives to maintain upper body strength. By learning early, they'll be that much ahead of the game.

Getting Ready

To do a push-up, lie face down with your arms shoulder-width apart, arms straight with your hands supporting you, head in line with your spine, and toes on the ground. Keeping your back straight, gently lower your upper body so that your elbows are bent at 90-degree angles and the upper arms are parallel to the floor. Slowly return to the straight-arm position.

A push-up sounds easy enough, but it's not. If your child can't get off the ground, start with much easier wall push-ups; once she can do them continuously for 60 seconds, move to the modified push-up. To do a wall push-up, stand facing a wall, holding your arms straight, shoulder's width apart, with your palms against the wall. Lean into the wall, bending your arms (if you have to move your feet you're too far from the wall). Push away from the wall to return to the starting position. That's a wall push-up.

A modified push-up is just like a regular push-up except that both your toes *and* your knees contact the ground. You still need to keep your back straight and your buttocks down, but this format is much easier than a regular push-up.

Allow your child to practice push-ups for a couple of weeks before you test her. She'll be surprised how quickly she can build her strength if she keeps at it.

22

What You Need

All you need to do a push-up is a firm, level surface and a willing child. That's why this exercise is so great. It can be done anytime, anywhere.

Doing the Test

Ask your child to get into position to do a push-up, starting with elbows straight. A complete push-up is when she lowers herself so her elbows are at 90 degrees and then returns to the starting position. She should try to do a push-up about every three seconds in a rhythmic fashion. If she hesitates for more than five seconds or so, the test is over. See Table 2.3 for scoring.

Table 2.3		Push-up Standards for Strength			
Boys			**Girls**		
Age	Fit	Needs to improve	Age	Fit	Needs to improve
5	3–8	<3	5	3–8	<3
6	3–8	<3	6	3–8	<3
7	4–10	<4	7	4–10	<4
8	5–13	<5	8	5–13	<5
9	6–15	<6	9	6–15	<6
10	7–20	<7	10	7–15	<7
11	8–20	<8	11	7–15	<7
12	10–20	<10	12	7–15	<7
13	12–25	<12	13	7–15	<7
14	14–30	<14	14	7–15	<7
15	16–35	<16	15	7–15	<7
16	18–35	<18	16	7–15	<7
17	18–35	<18	17	7–15	<7
17+	18–35	<18	17+	7–15	<7

Testing Strength and Flexibility

The trunk extensor test measures how well the abdominal muscles, hamstrings, and back extensor muscles work in concert. When these muscles are strong and flexible, your child has a reduced risk of back injury.

Getting Ready

Stretching his muscles regularly keeps your child agile and reduces his risk of a number of injuries. But a muscle that hasn't been worked lately should never be stretched. After a gentle workout or play period, encourage your child to perform a variety of stretches. The trunk extensor exercise can easily be practiced while watching TV or lying on the floor playing games.

What You Need

Your child will need to lie on a comfortable surface, such as a carpeted floor or mat. Wood or concrete floors are too uncomfortable, and beds and couches are too bouncy. You'll also need a yardstick.

Doing the Test

Have your child lie on his stomach with toes pointed behind him and hands straight by his sides. Have him lift his upper body off the ground very slowly to a maximum height of 12 inches (going any higher puts too much stress on the back). Place the ruler about an inch in front of your child's chin and measure how high he can get. Do not encourage him to bounce. Let him try again to see if he can go higher. Record the better of the two scores (see Table 2.4).

Table 2.4 Trunk-Lift Standards for Strength and Flexibility					
Boys			**Girls**		
Age	Fit	Needs to improve	Age	Fit	Needs to improve
5	6–12	<6	5	6–12	<6
6	6–12	<6	6	6–12	<6
7	6–12	<6	7	6–12	<6
8	6–12	<6	8	6–12	<6
9	6–12	<6	9	6–12	<6
10	9–12	<9	10	9–12	<9
11	9–12	<9	11	9–12	<9
12	9–12	<9	12	9–12	<9
13	9–12	<9	13	9–12	<9
14	9–12	<9	14	9–12	<9
15	9–12	<9	15	9–12	<9
16	9–12	<9	16	9–12	<9
17	9–12	<9	17	9–12	<9
17+	9–12	<9	17+	9–12	<9

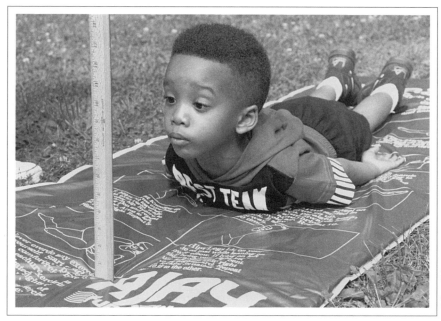

© Karen Maier

Measuring Flexibility

In the old days, being flexible was a "girl" thing. Ballerinas were flexible. Gymnasts like Cathy Rigby were flexible. But he-men, like football players, hockey stars, and body builders, weren't flexible, and that was okay. But now we know that everyone should be able to move their joints through an entire range of motions to avoid injuries and perform sports and chores more easily—even football players, hockey stars, and body builders. Real men stretch!

Did You Know?

Girls generally are more flexible than boys. The ability to bend is affected by hormones, and the ability to touch the toes is partly due to flexibility and also to body proportions.

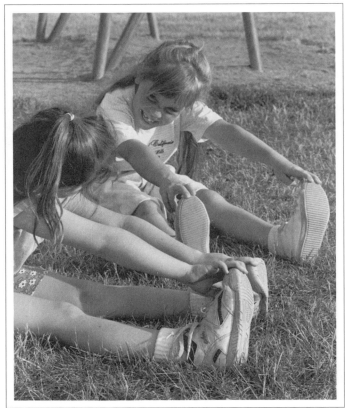

© Karen Maier

Getting Ready

The more you stretch, the more flexible you become. (Training is specific.) Always warm up a bit with some light exercise before you stretch or you could hurt yourself. This test checks your child's hamstring muscle flexibility. Being flexible other places is important, too, but these areas are easy, common markers for total-body flexibility. Before you test your child, encourage her to practice for a few weeks. Basic toe touches will do. But if you have the time and inclination, you can work together on a variety of stretches. Stretching is one fitness activity that parents can easily perform with their children. Often, in fact, your child will do better than you do!

What You Need

You will need a sturdy box or a stairstep about 12 inches high. Get a ruler that is between 18 and 24 inches long or make one out of stiff cardboard.

Place it so the 9-inch mark is exactly in line with the vertical plane of the edge of the box or step and the 1-inch mark is closest to your child. Tape it in place with strong clear packaging tape.

Doing the Test

After your child is warmed up a bit, have him take off his shoes and gently stretch out before the test. He can practice by touching his toes or reaching to the sky or around to his back with his arms. Once he feels limber, have him sit facing the step. One leg should be extended in front, with heel flat against the step or box; the other leg can be bent comfortably, with the sole of the foot on the ground. Hands are turned palms down on top of each other and stretched toward the end of the ruler. Let him reach forward slowly a couple of times to get good positioning. He shouldn't bounce when he reaches. If need be, place your hand on the knee of his straight leg so it doesn't bend. For testing, have him reach forward slowly as far as he can. Have your child hold the farthest position for 1 second and mark it. That's his score, calculated to the nearest half inch (see Table 2.5).

Table 2.5 Sit-and-Reach Standards for Flexibility					
Boys			**Girls**		
Age	Fit	Needs to improve	Age	Fit	Needs to improve
5	8	<8	5	9	<9
6	8	<8	6	9	<9
7	8	<8	7	9	<9
8	8	<8	8	9	<9
9	8	<8	9	9	<9
10	8	<8	10	9	<9
11	8	<8	11	10	<10
12	8	<8	12	10	<10
13	8	<8	13	10	<10
14	8	<8	14	10	<10
15	8	<8	15	12	<12
16	8	<8	16	12	<12
17	8	<8	17	12	<12
17+	8	<8	17+	12	<12

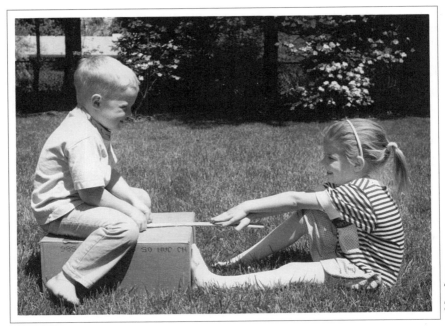

© Doug Brown

Measuring Body Composition

Knowing one's percentage of body fat is very useful in gauging fitness. Most height and weight charts, though, do not take body composition into account. Children with bigger bones or strong muscles may be labeled fat when they aren't. And slight children can look underweight when actually they are right on target. Even children who fall within the norms on a height and weight chart could be too fat.

There are a number of ways to measure body fat; unfortunately none are very easy to perform. Underwater weighing, the standard for body composition measurements, is usually done only at research facilities.

> **T**here is no such thing as a "perfect" body—no matter how hard you try. On the other hand, though, everyone can become fit and healthy, which should be enough.
>
> **Richard Simmons**
> *fitness instructor*

Most of the gizmos that measure body composition (calipers, bioelectrical impedance equipment, or near-infrared spectrophotometry) or the formulas (circumference girth measurements) have an error range of 3% to 6%, depending on the method and device used (and who is using the device). So if, for example, your child's physical educator tells you that your child has 18% body fat, it could actually be anywhere from 12% to 24%, including the error range. What does this mean? No measurement should be considered the gold standard. Instead, use the numbers you have as a baseline to monitor change (see Table 2.6).

Table 2.6 Percent-Fat Standards for Body Composition					
Boys			**Girls**		
Age	Good	Too high	Age	Good	Too high
5	14.7–20	>20	5	16.2–21	>21
6	14.7–20	>20	6	16.2–21	>21
7	14.9–20	>20	7	16.2–22	>22
8	15.1–20	>20	8	16.2–22	>22
9	15.2–20	>20	9	16.2–23	>23
10	15.3–21	>21	10	16.6–23.5	>23.5
11	15.8–21	>21	11	16.9–24	>24
12	16.0–22	>22	12	16.9–24.5	>24.5
13	16.6–23	>23	13	17.5–24.5	>24.5
14	17.5–24.5	>24.5	14	17.5–25	>25
15	18.1–25	>25	15	17.5–25	>25
16	18.5–25	>25	16	17.5–25	>25
17	18.8–27	>27	17	17.5–26	>26
17+	19–27.8	>27.8	17+	18–27.3	>27.3

If you are told your child has 18% body fat when he or she is 10 and each subsequent year it is similar or slightly higher, you can assume your child has a healthy body composition. However, a child who started with 18% at age 10 and by high school has 28% is putting on too much fat and should eat less fat and get more exercise.

It is imperative that calipers or circumference girth measurements are done by skilled professionals, because the margin of error is related to how well the measurements are taken. Errors from near-infrared spectrophotometry, on the other hand, are more likely to come from the instrument than the technician.

Many health clubs provide body fat measurements free or at low cost for members. Most professionals with degrees in exercise science or who are certified exercise specialists are trained to take measurements. Your child's physical education teacher may be able to take an accurate reading; likewise many nutritionists are skilled in this area. If you can't find someone to take an accurate measurement, ask your doctor for a referral.

Did You Know?

Most insurance guidelines for how much a woman or man of a given height should weigh are not accurate. Most such recommendations are based on what people weigh at death. However, many chronic diseases, such as cancer, often cause weight loss.

Be Warned: Fitness Testing Isn't Absolute

Absolutes can be so nice. Two plus two is always four. And the earth will always be round. Wouldn't it be nice to perform a battery of tests to determine exactly how fit you are and exactly what, if anything, you need to do to get better? It sounds too good to be true, and it is. Fitness and health promotion are not absolute. And, quite obviously, neither is a child's development.

Exercise science is still too new for researchers to be able to tell you firmly how fit your child is. How fat is too fat? How strong is strong enough? How will a child's current fitness level affect adult health? Scientists just haven't had the chance to thoroughly study what parameters in a child affect today's and tomorrow's fitness and health status.

Children also develop at vastly different speeds. Your child may be 10 years old, but he may have a body comparable to a 9-year-old today and a 10-year-old in a month. And that's okay! We want our children to be healthy and fit, no matter what their stages of development. Most fitness tests compare children by ages. Because children are still growing, this can be unfair to the late bloomer (who may seem weak and drop out of sports because of perceived failures) and the early bloomer (who may think sports should always be "easy" and later drops out when peers "catch up" and staying competitive gets tougher).

And children aren't necessarily the most reasonable creatures. At times you can't coax a bored child to move an inch, while that same child may run herself silly when she's out with her friends. Many fitness tests ask you to work out until exhaustion, which only a motivated child will do. A test isn't accurate if it isn't done correctly.

> ne of my greatest moments in my quest for fitness was when I learned a new skill that I hadn't been physically strong enough to do before. It felt good that I had been able to address a weak point in my training and improve on it.
>
> Kim Zemeskal
> *Olympic gymnast*

The standards from the Prudential Fitnessgram are quite wide-ranging; they allow for variance in physical development. Ideally, you would want your child performing at the upper levels of these standards, but the most important result is change. Did your child get quicker, stronger, leaner, or more flexible? Assessing your child's performance over time is the best way to use these numbers. Keep a log to record your child's results, and compare them at the next testing. Use the log we've included in this book (see Form 2.1), or send $2.50 to Prudential FITNESSGRAM, The Cooper Institute of Aerobics Research, 12330 Preston Rd., Dallas, TX 75280 (ph. 214-701-8001). And be sure to reward your child for improvement!

Now that you have a handle on how fit your child is, let's take the next step—helping your child be *more* fit.

Form 2.1		Log Sheet for Annual Test Results				
Physical Fitness Progression Log						
Year	1-Mile run	Body composition	Curl-up	Trunk lift	Modified pull-up	Sit-and-reach

Page 17 "Who Should conduct the Test?" through page 30, first paragraph, are reprinted from The Prudential FITNESSGRAM (1992).

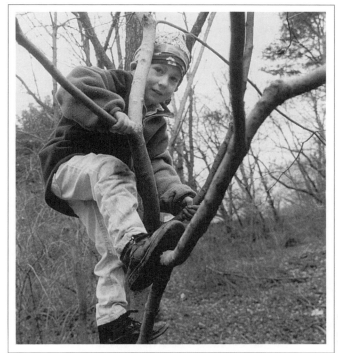

© Doug Brown

Helping Your
Child Get Fit

People who are avid exercisers sometimes have a hard time containing their enthusiasm. It's not that they want to preach but, frankly, they get so much out of their workouts that they want to help others experience the same type of rewards. Another group of people usually quite committed to their cause is parents. Most parents focus their priorities on their family.

If you put the two together—an avid exerciser who is a parent—the sum can be a very enthusiastic individual who pulls out all stops to get a child involved in sports. My son received his first baseball glove the day after he was born. He got a soccer ball before he could walk. These family gifts were well intentioned but inappropriate. Had the trend continued, my poor son would have amassed a storehouse of sporting goods that he was unprepared to use. Luckily we learned as our son mastered new skills and developed new interests to present appropriate new games, skills, and equipment.

In this chapter I'll talk a little about what you can expect physically and emotionally from children at various ages, then get down to the basics of training and sport selection.

Developmental Levels and Fitness

Your child's developmental age is not the same as her chronological age. Dr. Ken Cooper, the father of the fitness movement, in his book *Kid Fitness*, has outlined these developmental stages and tips to help your child. The years he suggests are based on averages. Every child is an experiment of one; your child may reach these milestones a little before or a little after indicated.

Phase 1—Starting From Scratch (The First Two Years)

At this early age start by building your child's self-confidence and curiosity. Praise and encourage her movements. Place her in settings where she can interact with her environment (away from dangerous objects and activities that encourage you to say no).

Start early with sound nutritional habits. Babies are the best judges of their caloric requirements. Feed your child when he is hungry. Never force or encourage him to eat when he is not. Don't use food as a reward or to quiet a child. If you use food as nourishment, not a treat, your child will develop a healthy attitude and appetite.

Phase 2—Beginning Skills (2–5 Years)

Once your child is relatively mobile and verbal (by age 2 or so), she is ready to learn about the wonderful world of physical activity. Learning basic skills at a young age is key for successful athletic performance later.

Did You Know?

A child who walks easily before age 1 won't necessarily be a star athlete, but walking is a sign of good balance and coordination.

Throwing, kicking, and jumping skills are the first skills learned. Children's boundless energy and willingness to please make them wonderful pupils. And their endless enthusiasm makes them repeat a newfound skill until they have it right . . . or until they are encouraged to try another new trick.

Don't worry if you're not very talented yourself. Just go over basic skills (see Table 3.1) with your child at his level, not yours. (And I must admit,

Table 3.1 Skills to Introduce to Pre-Schoolers*	
Controlling objects	
Catching	Dribbling
Hitting a ball with a bat or racket	Kicking
Punting	Throwing overhand
Throwing underhand	Trapping a ball with feet
Moving	
Balancing on one foot or a narrow surface	Galloping or skipping
Hopping on one foot	Jumping over something
Leaping or bounding forward	Riding a two-wheel bike
Running	Skipping
Sliding on ice or with rollar skates	Doing somersaults (front or back)
Strength	
Lifting	Pushing
Pulling	

*By 5 or 6 years of age, most children will be able to perform these skills on a basic level.
Adapted from Cooper (1991).

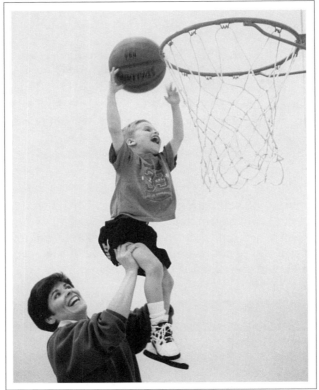

© Doug Brown

as I have practiced basic ball skills with my child, my throwing, kicking, and catching have improved too. It's never too late to work on the basics!) Your goal is to help your child understand the basics and to find enjoyment and confidence in executing them. Always present skills in a fun environment without being judgmental (except in a positive way).

Aside from these physical skills, your child should be able to follow directions, understand basic rules for games, and play thoughtfully with other children. She should also be able to report back to you about what she did and how she felt about it to help you monitor the fun factor when you're not around.

Phase 3—Being Active Just for the Heck of It (5–8 Years)

Children between the ages of about 5 and 8 play sports and exercise because it seems like the natural thing to do. They don't care much about winning. They care even less about strategy. Although they want to improve their skills, they aren't necessarily doing it to please you (as they are in the skill-building phase between ages 2 and 5). At this age, sport is more for companionship: to have fun, be with friends, and burn off energy, in that order. Goals for your child at this stage should center on improving fitness, providing adequate time and space to be as active as possible, and improving skills. It's okay for your child to sign up for a team sport at this age, as long as it's not winning-oriented or too structured.

Watch out for accidents. The confidence and skills developed in the last phase encourage risk taking in this one. Your child also is trying to exert more independence, so may be less responsive to your supervision. Set boundaries and explain cause-and-effect situations, but don't be overprotective. Provide as much latitude as you can within the boundaries you have set so your child's confidence in her movements continues to grow. Have a good first aid kit on hand.

Between ages 5 and 8 children are able to integrate physical and cognitive skills. After kicking the ball, they will begin naturally to follow it. After catching the ball, they will spontaneously throw it back. Called "spontaneous cueing," this is the first in a series of important mind-body developments that will allow your child to enjoy sports and improve his self-confidence.

Phase 4—Playing on a Team (8–10 Years)

A child who is about 8 or 9 is ready to begin playing team sports. Not only have they developed enough physical skills, they are still unself-conscious enough to try things they haven't yet mastered. And children this age can play by the rules. They still aren't too good at looking at the big picture (seeing how each player fits into the team), but they know enough to get out there, be a team player, and have fun.

Your main role at this stage is to help your child enjoy a variety of activities with friends—either playing team sports like basketball, soccer, and volleyball or participating in more individual activities like martial arts, aerobics, and swimming. Because there are wide variations in muscle strength, endurance, and height among children from age 8 through puberty, now is the time to ensure that your child is playing in environments that will encourage involvement and foster a positive self-image. Is your child ready physically, mentally, or socially for the activities? Encourage your child to be the best he can be, not better than your neighbor's child.

> **O**ne of my toughest obstacles when I was about 12 or 13 was that I felt I was clumsy. But through sports I improved my coordination and my image of myself.
>
> Bonnie Blair
> *Olympic speed skater*

Phase 5—Going Through Puberty (10–14 Years)

Puberty is a troubling time for many families. In fitness, however, if puberty is handled correctly, it can be a time of triumph, with earlier hard work coming together for success, fun, and long-term profit.

The trick is recognizing not just when children are going through puberty, but also what stage they are in and how we can help. Children begin puberty between the ages of 10 and 14 and can continue until age 18, though they have usually finished by age 16. Because puberty doesn't follow a set course, the uneven development between children mentioned in Phase 4 becomes obvious. Your number one concern at this age is to be absolutely sure that your child has access to playing sports with others who are at his stage in development of motor skills, endurance, and social abilities. Every molehill seems like a mountain during puberty. Don't augment the problem by letting your child get into environments where he will undoubtedly fail. A foul taste of fitness at this age can last a lifetime.

Boys are at a competitive disadvantage against peers who are more physically developed. They have less muscle mass and possibly coordination. Aside from looking for programs that match development rather than age, you may want your son to try sports that focus on personal development, such as martial arts, bicycling, hiking, and canoeing.

Girls are at more of a competitive disadvantage after puberty against girls who have not physically matured yet. As body fat and height increase, coordination and self-esteem may be affected. Help your daughter understand that increases in body fat during puberty are natural. A girl puts on body fat now to prepare for childbearing later in life. If she has been regular in her fitness endeavors, she will quickly regain any loss in self-image.

Be watchful of her getting too thin at this stage too. An unhealthy body image or low self-esteem, coupled with the mild increase in body fat, may cause the development of an eating disorder that causes your daughter to try to maintain too little body fat. I'll discuss this more in chapter 4. If you are concerned about your daughter's low body fat, talk with her doctor.

Phase 6—Almost an Adult (14–17 Years)

After puberty, your child has almost developed the body of an adult (though with more hair and fewer wrinkles). The self-image established in previous years is now firmly in place. If you did your job, it's a good one. If you didn't, you can still help your son or daughter to embrace fitness, but it's harder.

Begin refocusing fitness goals on long-term benefits. Your child is beginning to look at how he plans to enter adulthood. Help him see where exercise and sports play a role. Most high schools do not require physical education for students. Either be sure your child takes advantage of existing programs or look for extracurricular programs at community and recreation centers.

Now is the time to discuss the hows and whys of fitness education. It's a key to helping your teen take responsibility for her health. Make sure she has access to good books and videos on diet, training, and injury prevention. Discuss training, responsibility, and fitness with her regularly.

> **P**arents need to instill in their children an honor system that integrates athletic competition and the real world.
>
> **Jon Stevenson**
> *professional volleyball player*

Getting Fit

Now that you have a better idea of what to expect from your child as well as of his strengths and weaknesses, it's time to get to the sweat of the matter. Keep these key principles in mind.

▼ Together with your child you can set a fitness goal and map out a program to progress slowly and attain it. By gradually increasing how hard, how long, or how many times he does an exercise or drill, your child will improve. It takes 6 to 8 weeks to notice most fitness improvements, so be patient. Try plotting out the program on a calendar and crossing off the workouts. That way your child can see the progress on the calendar even if he doesn't see it on his body. If your child does too much too fast, he can develop a sports injury or burn out or get bored and turn away from sports.

▼ Your child needs to work out regularly. Whether it's once, twice, or ideally 3 to 5 times a week, training regularly brings results. Regularity also breeds habit.

▼ Getting better means trying harder. Your child should push himself to improve by trying to run longer, throw farther, swim faster. As the heart and other muscles are forced to work harder, they become stronger. After the next exercise session (if muscles are rested), the muscles can do that much again, and probably more.

▼ Training is specific. To make baskets, your child must practice shooting. To land soccer goals, she must practice kicking. To run faster, she must practice running fast.

With these principles in mind, let's look back at the basic components of fitness.

Building Endurance

While some sports, such as running, biking, and swimming, improve your child's endurance just by doing them, others, such as basketball, baseball, and downhill skiing, don't help as much. The best ways to improve endurance are to run, walk, swim, bike, aerobic dance, cross-country ski, skate, hike, jump rope, and dance. Fun team sports that build endurance include soccer, field hockey, ice hockey, and lacrosse.

Do one of these activities or a combination—called cross-training—3 or 4 times a week. Alternate hard and easy days so that the body has a chance to rest, recover, and come back stronger than ever. To increase endurance, gradually extend each long session by 5 or 10 minutes. Once every 3 or 4 weeks, go the distance. Take a nice long hike or bike ride with your child, or do something moderately vigorous for a couple of hours. These endurance sessions will keep you in top form, with the stamina to have fun at almost any activity.

Exercise at a constant intensity so that you keep moving for 15 to 20 minutes without stopping. If you get too tired before the time is up, no matter how slowly you go, alternate your activity with increments of rest, walking, or gliding. For example, after 3 minutes of pedaling, glide for

30 seconds, then repeat the cycle. Gradually reduce the time you spend combining low-intensity activity with a faster-paced activity until you can do the entire 15- or 20-minute workout without stopping.

Don't coax your child with negative words if he can't keep up ("Hey, slow poke—I can't believe you're tired already!"). Usually a child who is having fun will be giving his all. Instead, look for ways to make the activity more fun. Play tag or chase (and let him catch you sometimes). Change the activity often—after kicking the ball around for a while, take off and run around the field, try to touch the top of the goal post, then play Pickle in the Middle.

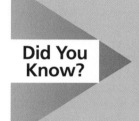

Did You Know?

Cross-country skiing is a great fitness workout for the whole body. It strengthens muscles, builds endurance and flexibility, and works both the upper and lower body. It's also a great fat burner.

Building Strength

You can do specific exercises to improve your strength, such as crunches and wall sits. Aspects of specific sports, such as running on hills, also increase strength. Here are a few exercises that, if done a couple of times a week, will ensure that you become stronger. Try these out yourself, then show your child.

Crunch

Lie on your back with knees bent and feet on the floor. Cross your hands over your chest, then curl up so that your head and shoulders are off the ground and you are raised about 30 degrees. Your stomach muscles should feel tight. Slowly lower yourself back to the starting position. Once you can do 10 repetitions, increase by increments of 5 until you can do them continuously for 60 seconds.

Heel Raise

Holding onto the rail for balance, stand on a step and hang your heels over the edge. Raise your heels as far as possible and hold for 1 or 2 seconds—your calf muscles should feel tight. Slowly return to the starting position. Once you can do 10 repetitions, increase by increments of 5 until you can do 50 at once.

Wall Jump

Stand sideways next to a wall and reach up. Mark (mentally or with a piece of tape) a spot on the wall 1 yard above your fingers. Drop the arm, bend your knees, and leap up to try to touch the mark. Repeat 10 times on each side.

Modified Pull-Up

It is important that your child be able to lift his own weight. In case of a fire or accident, your child may need to climb out of a window or car, using mostly upper body strength. Most girls over age 12 can't hang on for dear life for very long. Few boys over age 16 can lower themselves down a rope easily. By practicing pull-ups or modified pull-ups your child will be more able to get out of a tight spot. Because most children can't do pull-ups, do a modified pull-up.

Place a strong pole or pipe (about 6 feet long) across the seats of two chairs placed about 3 feet apart. The chairs should be sturdy and heavy enough that they won't tip over. Secure the bar with a rope or strong adhesive tape (I always use duct tape). Lie on your back, slide under the bar, and grasp it with two hands, palms facing away from your body and hands about shoulder-width apart. Pull your chest up to the bar keeping your body straight from head to toe. Do this 10 times. The easier this gets, the higher the bar can be raised (the use of a doorway pull-up bar makes this easier). Eventually you can work your way up to a bar high enough that your body hangs completely off the ground.

Becoming More Flexible

Simple stretching exercises increase flexibility. Warm up your muscles before stretching by doing enough aerobic activity to break a sweat, or stretch at the end of a workout. Don't bounce when stretching, and never stretch to the point of pain. Gradually move into your stretches—don't jerk or race through them. Hold each stretch 15 to 30 seconds.

Back Reach

Raise your right hand in the air with palm facing to the back. Bend your elbow and place your palm between your shoulders. Bring your left hand behind your back and try to touch your right hand. Hold and repeat on the other side.

Groin Stretch

Sit on the floor with your legs bent and the soles of your feet together. Gently press your knees toward the floor using your hands until the muscles in your inner thighs become tense.

Hip Flexor Stretch

Lying on your back, use your arms to pull one leg up tight to the chest while the other leg stays slightly bent in front of you. Return your leg to the starting position and repeat on the other side.

Hamstrings Stretch (Back of the Thigh)

Sitting on the floor with your legs straight ahead and your knees slightly bent, bend forward and reach to your toes.

Quadriceps Stretch (Front of the Thigh)

Lie on your left side and bend your right knee so the foot is behind you. Grab your right foot with your right hand. Gently pull back until the thigh muscles are tight and hold. Lie on your right side and repeat with the left leg.

Calf Stretch

Stand about arm's length from a wall and lean into the wall with arms outstretched. Slide one foot back a foot or two, keeping both heels on the floor. Bend the forward leg and lean forward until you feel a stretch in the calf of the back leg. In that same position, slightly bend the back leg, hold, then straighten the back leg. Hold again. Return to the original position and change legs.

> **I** either undertrained or overtrained. Balance is key to both sports and life. Sometimes you need to sit back to be sure you are on the right track.
>
> Billie Jean King
> *professional tennis player*

Developing an Exercise Schedule

Most children will benefit from a loose program that allows them to play to improve their fitness levels. But keep these basic activity components in the back of your mind, especially if your child is working under the supervision of a coach.

You will want to be sure your child works out at least 4 times a week for 20 to 60 minutes a session, like adults are told to do. But, as you probably know all too well, children are innately active. Instead of scheduling workout sessions, plan for fitness activities. Remember to count recreation time at school (physical education class and recess), after school (community leagues, recreation centers, and backyard play), and with your family (sports play, yard work and housework, and roughhousing). Does your child walk home from school? That's a workout too. Your goal should be to make sure that your child builds up to a sweat and gets her heart racing for a least 4 or 5 hours a week. How that is broken down is up to your child's interests and your schedule.

Warm-Up

Before any strenuous activity your child should gently warm up muscles. In many cases that involves easy motions of the sport, such as gentle stretching, jogging, tossing the ball around—whatever he plans on doing later, but at a relaxed pace.

Cross-Training and Hard or Easy Days

To build endurance and strength requires stressing a muscle, then resting it. Usually the best way to do this is to work out hard one day and easier the next. Your child should avoid working the same muscle, and avoid doing the same sport, *hard* every day. People who cross-train (that is, do more than one sport) can alternate sports regularly so they don't work the same muscles daily.

Cool-Down

Your child should allow his body to gently cool down after a workout by doing the same routine he did when warming up or just walking around a bit until his heart stops racing. He should never just sit down after a very hard workout.

Regularity

Why should activity be regular? Because if you don't use it (be it strength, endurance, or a skill) you lose it—even children.

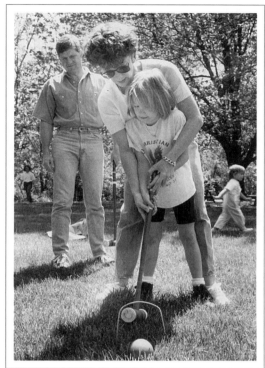

© Doug Brown

Getting Better

A child who wants to improve her skill in a certain activity needs to increase the frequency, duration, or intensity of her play. But don't let her increase all three areas at once. She can gradually increase frequency first (play an easy game of tennis 3 or 4 times a month), then look at the duration (lengthen her tennis time from one set to three or five a session), and then work on intensity (once she plays as often as she likes and for as long as she likes, she can start working on playing harder and refining her skill).

What if your child plays a team sport? Again, to improve he needs to practice. Generally, he should practice the skill formally with a coach or team once a week, practice informally by himself or with friends once or twice a week, and then use the skill in competition once a week.

With Pain, There Is No Gain

If an exercise hurts or your child finds a movement uncomfortable, something is wrong. The '80s exercise adage No pain, no gain is dead wrong. Often enthusiasm drives a child to start out at too high an intensity or to work out too often, increasing the risk of injury or burnout. Instead, exercise should be fun, and while it can be stressful, it shouldn't be painful.

Rest Is Important

After a muscle or bone is stressed, it will get stronger only if it is allowed to rest. The harder the stress, the more rest your child needs.

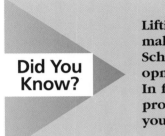

Did You Know?

Lifting weights regularly won't necessarily make you look like bodybuilder Arnold Schwarzenegger. That type of muscle development takes a specialized lifting regimen. In fact, lifting weights correctly often improves flexibility, firms muscles, and helps you maintain a healthy body composition.

Exercise Concerns

The more involved you become in your child's fitness, the more questions you may have. Here are answers to some of parents' most common questions.

Should Children Lift Weights?

Children benefit from building their strength, but in most cases they can do that through their sport or a drill rather than by lifting weights. If your child wants to lift weights or a coach recommends it, be sure she is supervised by a trained strength and conditioning specialist. She needs to be emotionally mature enough to follow directions carefully. Form is key when lifting; and it is important to lift the right amount of weight and perform the correct number of repetitions. A spotter, or assistant, should be there to help with the weights and to monitor safe lifting procedures.

Should Girls and Boys Play Sports Together?

Children should play with others who are at the same developmental level. Until age 8 or 9, boys and girls develop at about the same rate, and there is no reason they shouldn't play together. Beyond age 9, however, development, not gender, is key. Your child should play with peers of similar size and skill level. That can mean playing with girls or boys, older or younger. That said, many adolescent girls feel uncomfortable competing against boys. This attitude is often culturally based and supported by peers. Encourage your daughter's belief in her abilities so that she has the confidence to play in arenas with developmentally matched peers. But don't force your child into any competition.

Can a Child Overtrain?

If your child complains after a practice or a workout that he's too tired or sore to return, ask more about his feelings regarding his activities. Does he like the coach? Does he feel he's improving? Does he have fun at practice? If not, take steps to try to avoid a fitness dropout, or steer him to a sport or team he can enjoy more.

But if your child does enjoy her sport but is experiencing fatigue and soreness, she may be overtraining and on her way to an injury or burnout. Common signs of overtraining include

- fatigue, sluggishness, increased heart rate at rest,
- grumpiness and irritability,
- poor appetite,
- soreness and stiffness,
- frequent colds,
- heavy-feeling legs,
- poor sleep patterns, and
- seemingly constant thirst.

If you think your child may be overdoing it, contact his coach or physical education teacher and communicate your concerns. Let him miss practice or class for a week and see if he bounces back. If he doesn't, check with your pediatrician. Catch overtraining early, before your child burns out.

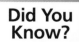

Did You Know?

Grumpy exercisers should check their training. Negative moods are often one of the first signs of overtraining.

Helping Your Young Superstar

So many people wish they could be elite athletes. Watching the Olympics gets most spectators dreaming. Elite athletes look so talented, so happy, so skilled. But being an elite child athlete is anything but easy. Elite child athletes can develop problems in a number of areas.

Family Relationships

Your child's training and competition schedules can disrupt family meals, vacations, and holidays. Siblings can feel left out if attention and family activities center on your athlete and her schedule. Be sensitive to the entire family. Is your child's involvement in sport worth disrupting the family? Try to develop family rituals that are not interrupted by sports.

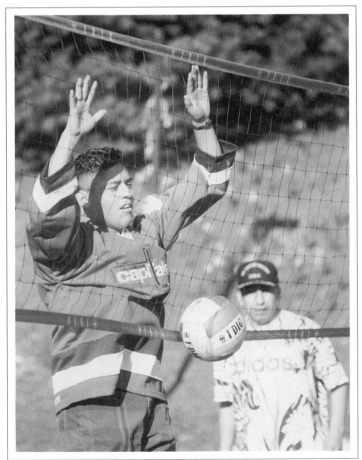

© Doug Brown

Social Relationships

Competitive young athletes often feel out of step with their peers. While they may have numerous friends from their sport or school, they still can feel different. Many times an athlete's body develops differently than his or her peers' do. And children, especially adolescents, don't want to be different. The amount of time an athlete devotes to his sport also makes it difficult for him to hang out with friends. I had a friend in high school whom I always admired; she was a gymnast in the Junior Olympics. At a reunion I told her how envious I was of her back then. She laughed and told me I was the lucky one. I had played sports throughout school, gotten good grades, and been able to go to football games and parties. By contrast, her grades were dismal and her social life was nil. In the long run, I guess I was the winner.

Coach Relationships

No one wants your child to improve more than you do, except maybe her coach. In some instances, a coach can step back and help a child develop into a gifted, well-rounded adult. In other cases, a coaching career may dominate the picture, and your child's best interest may not be the focus. Choosing a coach for your gifted child is as important as choosing a good doctor or a good school. Take your time. Educate yourself on what's available. Don't abdicate your responsibility to your child just because her coach knows her sport better. You know your child better!

Academics

Most elite child athletes cannot earn a living in their sports when they grow up. But even though parents, coaches, and sometimes even the athletes themselves know it, they still forgo their book learning and head for the gym. Don't let your child convince you it is OK to focus on short-term athletic achievements in lieu of academic excellence. Even a child who receives an athletic scholarship to college is very unlikely to compete professionally. And he may not even graduate from college, which is the whole point behind the scholarship. Georgetown University has had a nationally ranked basketball program for many years. But that doesn't stop Coach John Thompson from benching players for poor grades. There are a number of wonderful careers relating to sports that gifted athletes can pursue. Sports medicine, teaching, coaching, research, journalism, and retailing are all much more realistic options than professional sports. Don't let your child forget his books!

Behavior Problems

Many of the psychological attributes that help children be good athletes can also provoke dangerous or excessive behavior. The strong desire to win may encourage an athlete to do unhealthy things, such as take anabolic steroids to become stronger or cut food intake to dangerously low levels to lose weight. Elite competitive athletes have also been known to take unhealthy chances, binge, or exhibit other reckless behavior to counterbalance the intense discipline they live with. Emotional immaturity may also be a problem expressed through temper tantrums and outbreaks. Do not tolerate poor behavior from your child, no matter how gifted she may be in sports. Keep focusing on why sports are a part of your child's life—to enrich it.

Did You Know?

When asked if they would encourage their children to participate in sports, 40% of the former elite athletes polled said no, at least not at an elite level as they had participated.

The pressure to succeed drives many young athletes to forgo normal school experiences and social activities in lieu of rigorous training and competition schedules. Families who alter their lifestyles for these athletes increase the pressure on them to succeed. Few elite child athletes enjoy sports as adults. Why do so many young elite athletes drop out of sports? If it isn't due to injury, it's burnout. In most cases, the fun factor in sports has gotten lost.

These first three chapters have focused on physical activity as a key to physical fitness. But there's more. What your child puts in his mouth greatly affects his ability to perform both on and off the field. And good nutrition also affects his chances of not developing many life-threatening diseases. Chapter 4 will teach you about making healthy food choices.

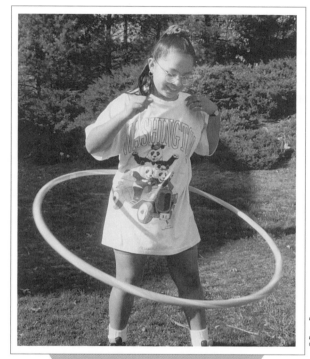

© Doug Brown

Food for Fitness

Eating habits, like many others, are learned early. Humans don't naturally crave sweets and fatty foods. These are yearnings we acquire from parents, peers, and society. I'll never forget a grocery shopping trip when my son was 3 years old. He came up to the cart carrying Lucky Charms cereal and told me how "magically delicious" they were and that he truly wanted to have some. Frankly, eating colored marshmallows first thing in the morning is a sensation I'd like to miss. Yet my son was convinced this was the greatest cereal—though he never had tasted it. Television commercials created his need.

If you have a high-performance car, the last thing you want to do is put bad fuel in it. The car will run, but its performance will suffer. The same goes for nutrition: Children who eat lots of fatty or processed foods, enjoy regular helpings of sweet desserts and candy, and don't get enough of the essential nutrients will still get around. But they won't feel as healthy as they could. And worse, they'll be inviting future health problems, including cancer and heart disease. Children's diet not only affects their energy level, it also helps prevent (or encourage) disease.

Parents as Key Players

If we lament our children's terrible eating habits, remember that they didn't crawl into a fast food restaurant for their first visit—someone took them. Choices we make affect the food choices our children will make in the future. Even so, many parents throw up their hands in disgust over food battles by the time a child is 2. "Jake won't eat vegetables," "Jenna will only drink chocolate milk," parents whimper in despair. Frankly, Jenna's and Jake's eating habits are a direct reflection of their parents' eating habits and what they allow their children to get away with.

One difference between kids who are served nutritious meals at home and kids who aren't is that the ones who are often believe nutritious foods taste good. Because they have tasted so many different healthful foods, these children have found some they truly like. American children over 2 years old eat exactly as the adults who raise them do. Stock your kitchen with nutritious food. What you don't purchase, your children won't eat.

Take the following quiz on how much fat you and your family eat to see how you stack up in this important area.

Do You Run a Fat Kitchen?

You have enormous control over what your family consumes at home. Are you helping your children learn to eat healthfully? Take this quiz to see if you are cutting the fat; answer each question, then total your points.

1. Do you plan ahead by purchasing or preparing lowfat snacks?
   a. never   b. occasionally   c. regularly

2. Do you read nutritional labels and use this information to select lowfat, nutritional foods?
   a. never   b. occasionally   c. regularly

3. What type of ice cream or frozen dessert do you buy for your family?
   a. gourmet   b. regular   c. light   d. sherbets

4. How often do you deep-fat fry food?
   a. never   b. occasionally   c. regularly

5. Do you put butter or margarine on vegetables before your serve them?
   a. never   b. occasionally   c. regularly

6. When you pan-fry foods, what type of oil do you use?
   a. I never pan-fry   b. butter or margarine   c. vegetable oil
   d. nonstick spray   e. olive or canola oil   f. shortening or lard

7. What percentage of the meals you serve are mostly homemade?
   a. less than 50% b. 50% to 75% c. 76% to 90% d. more than 90%

8. What type of milk do you serve at home?
   a. skim   b. 1%   c. 2%   d. whole

9. How often do you serve red meat each week?
   a. less than twice   b. 2 to 4 times   c. more than 4 times

10. How often does your family eat dessert?
    a. never   b. occasionally   c. regularly

✓Scoring

1. a. 0   b. 2   c. 6

2. a. 0   b. 2   c. 4

3. a. 0   b. 1   c. 2   d. 3

4. a. 3   b. 0   c. –5

5. a. 3   b. 0   c. –3

6. a. 3   b. –2   c. 0   d. 2   e. 1   f. –2

7. a. –2   b. 0   c. 1   d. 3

8. a. 3   b. 2   c. 1   d. 0

9. a. 3   b. 2   c. –1

10. a. 1   b. 1   c. –1

✓Results

More than 14—You're doing a great job providing your family with lowfat options.

4 to 14—Look for more lowfat alternatives.

Under 4—Your child doesn't have a good shot at establishing a lowfat diet because you aren't keeping fat out of the food choices you make. Use the information in this chapter to start changing your habits.

Elements of a Good Diet

Youngsters have a greater need than adults for nutrients and calories. A healthful diet contains the following elements: fat, carbohydrates, protein, vitamins, minerals, and water.

Fat

Fat is the primary source of stored energy, used during low-energy activities like eating, sleeping, and reading. Most Americans eat too much fat. Total fat intake should be at most 25% to 30% of your child's calories. The average American child gets 38% of calories from fat.

Not all fat is created equal. Animal fats, found in butter, meat, and milk, are primarily saturated. Tropical oils and hydrogenated fats are also saturated. Studies show that if you consume too much fat, especially saturated fat, you increase your risk of heart disease and cancer—at any age! Vegetable fats, found in oils from plant sources, are usually polyunsaturated. This type of fat isn't so bad for you.

Your first choice should be monounsaturated fats, found in olive and canola oils. They have been found to be less harmful than polyunsaturated and saturated fats. In some cases, they can actually be beneficial.

Reduce Fat in Your Family's Diet

We acquire preferences for what we typically eat. The more fatty foods your kids eat, the more they will prefer fatty foods. Even eating foods made from fat substitutes (nonfat mayonnaise, for example) keeps the taste of fat on the palate. By slowly cutting back on the fats in your diet, you will learn to prefer lowfat foods. Here are some tips:

- Use fats and oils sparingly in cooking. Bake, grill, poach, steam, and broil instead of deep frying or sautéing. Use nonstick vegetable oil sprays to reduce cooking fat.

- Use lowfat versions of milk, yogurt, and cheese.

- Peanut butter, a staple of most children's diets, is loaded with fat. Don't gob it on the bread—spread a thin layer instead, and be more generous with preserves, jams, and fresh fruits.

- Use small amounts of salad dressing and spreads such as butter, margarine, and mayonnaise. Try reduced-fat or nonfat substitutes.

- Before buying processed foods, check the labels for fat content. Choose products that have less than a third of their calories from fat.

- When preparing macaroni and cheese, stuffing, or sauces from packaged mixes, use only half the fat suggested. If milk or cream is called for, use lowfat milk.

Did You Know?

The best way to reduce the cholesterol in your blood is to cut the fat in your diet. Cutting cholesterol isn't as important as cutting fat.

Cholesterol

Diet also affects health by affecting cholesterol levels in the blood. Thirty years ago no one seemed to know what cholesterol was. Now we're not only talking about it, we've even labeled some cholesterol good and some bad! Studies have found that many children have dangerously high levels of cholesterol. While children won't die from this condition, they usually grow up to be adults with the same problem. And adults with high cholesterol levels have an increased risk of heart disease and stroke. (See Table 4.1 for cholesterol levels rated for children.)

Table 4.1 Total Cholesterol Levels for Children	
Risk level	**Cholesterol (milligrams per deciliter)**
Healthy	<169
Moderate risk	170–185
High risk	186–200
Very high risk	>200

Reprinted from Cooper (1991).

If your child has a moderate level of cholesterol in her blood, your doctor will probably prescribe a lowfat diet. People who consume fewer than 30% of their calories from fat, and only 10% from saturated fats, are much less likely to have cholesterol problems. If this strategy doesn't work, a more drastic diet is recommended. Children with cholesterol levels above 200 mg/dl (milligrams per deciliter—the standard way of expressing blood cholesterol) or who have a family history of heart disease or stroke are supervised closely by their doctors, and drug therapy may be recommended.

Although diet affects your child's cholesterol level, his activity, in part, also affects his level of high-density lipoprotein cholesterol (HDL-C, the "good cholesterol" that acts as a street sweeper, rounding up bad cholesterol and helping to get it out of the body). To get an even better picture of patients' health risks, doctors divide the amount of good cholesterol into the total cholesterol amount to find a "ratio" of good to total. That is, if total cholesterol is 180 and HDL-C is 39, the cholesterol ratio is 4.6 (180 ÷ 39). Table 4.2 lists healthy cholesterol ratios for children before and after puberty.

Table 4.2 Healthy Cholesterol Ratios for Children		
Risk Level	**Boys**	**Girls**
Before puberty		
Healthy	<2:9	<3:1
Moderate risk	2:9–3:3	3:1–3:4
High risk	3:4–3:5	3:5–3:7
Very high risk	>3:5	>3:7
After puberty		
Healthy	<3:7	<2:9
Moderate risk	3:7–5:1	2:9–3:6
High risk	5:2–6:1	3:7–4:2
Very high risk	>6:1	>4:2

Reprinted from Cooper (1991).

Doctors determine cholesterol levels through blood tests. The American Academy of Pediatrics recommends that before age 6, only children with a family history of heart disease or high blood cholesterol need to have their cholesterol checked. After age 6, your child should be checked every other year unless symptoms develop.

Carbohydrates

Carbohydrates are also an important fuel source, especially during exercise. If you are like most Americans, you're not eating enough carbohydrates. Between 60% and 65% of your total calories should come from carbohydrates, such as fruits, vegetables, breads, and grains.

Dietary fiber is basically a type of complex carbohydrate made up of plant material that cannot be digested by the human body. Refining and processing foods removes almost all of their natural fiber. The main sources of dietary fiber are fruits, vegetables, and whole-grain cereals and breads. Optimal amounts of fiber in the diet promote regular bowel movements and lower blood cholesterol, and may thus reduce the incidence of diverticulitis, colon and rectum cancer, and heart disease.

Research suggests that people who consume significant amounts of "cruciferous" vegetables (such as broccoli, cabbage, cauliflower, brussels sprouts, bok choy, collards, kale, kohlrabi, and mustard greens) tend to have lower cancer rates. By calling broccoli "trees" or stir-frying cabbage with your child's favorite meat, you can package a potentially unpopular food so that it looks and tastes like a winner. Be creative.

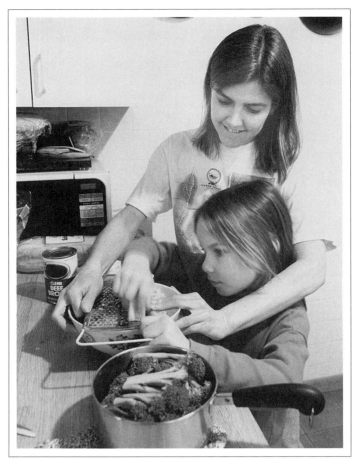

© Doug Brown

Protein

Although protein can be used for fuel, its primary purposes are to build and repair muscles, hair, and other tissues and to synthesize hormones. Most Americans consume too much protein. About 12% to 15% of your total calories should come from protein, which is found in meat, fish, and legumes, such as dried beans.

If you're the typical eater, you get most of your protein from red meat. But this source of protein contains too much saturated fat to be eaten regularly in a healthful diet. (Did you know that the average hot dog is almost 80% fat?)

Center your meals around alternatives to meat, like fish, beans, and pasta dishes. When you do serve meat, use only lean cuts, trim visible fat, and limit serving sizes to 4 ounces (about the size of a deck of cards).

Remove skin from chicken before cooking. If you send your child to school with meat sandwiches, choose thinly sliced chicken- or turkey-based meats. Avoid meats where you can see the fat, like salami.

Vitamins

Vitamins are not a source of energy. Rather, they work as catalysts to regulate the chemical reactions in your body. Vitamin C acts as an antioxidant, protecting your body from substances and chemical reactions that damage tissue. Some research suggests that vitamin C reduces the risk of colds and cancers. Vitamin E and beta-carotene also seem to act as antioxidants. Foods rich in these vitamins include citrus fruits, peppers, broccoli, tomatoes, strawberries, potatoes, apricots, peaches, cantaloupe, carrots, winter squashes, spinach, vegetable oils, whole grains, and wheat germ.

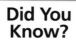

Did You Know?

Dark, colorful vegetables usually contain more nutrients than paler ones. Colorful broccoli, spinach, green peppers, tomatoes, and carrots have more nutritional value than celery, mushrooms, zucchini, cucumbers, and iceberg lettuce.

Minerals

Minerals, like vitamins, do not supply energy. But they help you develop structures in the body, like bones, and regulate body processes, like transporting oxygen. Important minerals include calcium, iron, magnesium, phosphorus, sodium, potassium, and zinc.

Topping the list of nutrients needed during childhood and adolescence is iron. Iron-deficiency anemia is the most common nutritional deficiency in the U.S. Iron is necessary to make red blood cells, among other functions. It is especially important for adolescent girls because of the onset of menstruation with its monthly blood losses.

Calcium is vital for building strong bones and teeth during childhood. Some experts believe that the recommended dietary allowance for calcium should be increased, especially for girls, because women are more prone to osteoporosis, and irreversible disease characterized by bone-thinning in later life. (The recommended dietary allowances of vitamins and minerals are the minimum amounts you need to prevent disease [see Table 4.3].) Researchers do not know how much of these nutrients are

Table 4.3	Recommended Dietary Allowances for Children			
Age	Protein (grams*)	Calcium (milligrams)	Iron (milligrams)	Calories
1–3	23	800	15	900–1,800
4–6	30	800	10	1,300–2,300
7–10	34	800	10	1,650–3,300
11–14 (boys)	45	1,200	18	2,000–3,700
11–14 (girls)	46	1,200	18	1,500–3,000
15–18 (boys)	56	1,200	18	2,100–3,900
15–18 (girls)	46	1,200	18	1,200–3,000

*One ounce equals about 28 grams.

Source: Food and Nutrition Board, National Academy of Sciences, National Research Council, 1980.

necessary to improve your health.) Osteoporosis can develop in people who consume too little calcium or do too little weight-bearing exercise in childhood. The best sources of calcium are milk products, but beware—dairy foods can be rich in fat, so choose lowfat varieties. Nondairy sources of calcium include bony fish (such as sardines and salmon), tofu, and spinach.

Should Children Take Vitamin Supplements?

This is a common question from parents, and often it's a hard one to answer. While your child is probably getting enough vitamins and minerals to avoid disease, it is not clear whether he is getting enough to promote good health. Research is not yet clear on what and how much is needed in this area. We do know, however, that nutrients are more readily absorbed if you get them from food rather than from pills.

With this in mind, it surely won't hurt if you give your child a daily multivitamin. Adolescent girls may benefit from vitamins fortified with iron and calcium. Some researchers recommend vitamin E be taken as a supplement because consuming enough to get an antioxidant protection would require large amounts of calories. However, adequate vitamin C and beta-carotene can be obtained through a carbohydrate-rich diet.

Did You Know? Caffeine reduces the body's ability to absorb iron. Children get caffeine in many soft drinks and in chocolate.

Water

Many people forget the importance of water, which makes up about two thirds of the body. Water stabilizes body temperature, carries nutrients to and waste away from cells, and helps the cells to function. Your children and you need to drink six to eight glasses of water a day. When you get thirsty, it means you've waited too long to drink. Thirst is not a good indicator of need. Urine color is a good sign—if urine is yellowish rather than nearly clear, more water is needed.

Salt

Children need about 1 to 3 grams of sodium (a component of salt) a day. Most get up to seven times that amount! Some people have a sensitivity that causes their blood pressure to rise when they eat salt. Your taste for salt is acquired. If you don't use much salt in your household, your children won't be as likely to want it. Many processed foods are filled with sodium, so read labels carefully if you're concerned about sodium intake.

Setting the Table for Health

Now that you know the basic components of a diet, how should you put them together? How much? How often? The U.S. Department of Agriculture has developed a food pyramid (see Figure 4.1) to outline what you should eat each day. It's not a rigid prescription but a basic guide that lets you put together a healthier diet for your family. In general, base meals on plenty of breads, cereals, rice, pasta, vegetables, and fruits. Complement these foods with a little meat, cheese, eggs, dried beans, or nuts. And only sparingly eat fats, oils, and sweets.

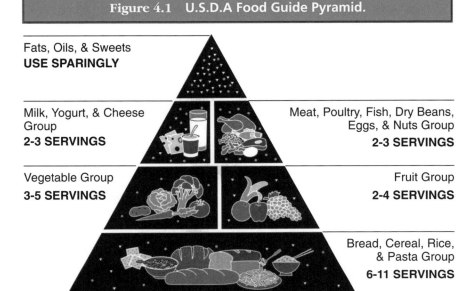

Figure 4.1 U.S.D.A Food Guide Pyramid.

Fats, Oils, & Sweets
USE SPARINGLY

Milk, Yogurt, & Cheese Group
2-3 SERVINGS

Meat, Poultry, Fish, Dry Beans, Eggs, & Nuts Group
2-3 SERVINGS

Vegetable Group
3-5 SERVINGS

Fruit Group
2-4 SERVINGS

Bread, Cereal, Rice, & Pasta Group
6-11 SERVINGS

Source: U.S. Department of Agriculture

What nutritionists consider a serving is not a hefty amount. Check out your dinner plate—how many "servings" do you really have? One serving is actually these amounts:

- 1/2 cup of fruit or vegetable
- 3/4 cup of juice
- 1 slice of bread
- 1 cup of milk

- 1 average piece of fruit
- 1 cup of salad greens
- 1/2 cup of cooked pasta
- Lean meat about the size of a deck of cards

See Table 4.4 to discover how many servings of which food groups your family members need.

Calorie requirements in childhood, especially in adolescence, vary widely with age, height, weight, and amount of physical activity. Children who are physically active need to be sure to eat enough to promote good growth and maturation.

Table 4.4 How Many Servings Does Your Family Need?			
Servings	Most women, all older adults	Children, teen girls, active women, most men	Teen boys, active men
Bread group	6	9	11
Vegetable group	3	4	5
Fruit group	2	3	4
Milk group	2*	2*	2*
Meat group	2	2	3

*Pregnant and breastfeeding women, teenagers, and anyone under age 24 need three milk group servings a day.

Source: U.S. Department of Agriculture

How Many Calories Should Your Child Consume?

Many parents ask how much—or how little—their child really needs to eat. For many kids, a Big Mac with cheese can cover half of their daily caloric needs, with little nutritional value. Here is a neat formula to use to help you estimate how many calories your child (or you!) need daily. Use the numbers as a guide; if you see undesirable changes in your child's weight, adjust the diet as needed.

1. Multiply your child's desired body weight by 10 to determine resting metabolic rate (the number of calories needed to maintain bodily functions).

2. To find out what additional calories are needed, start with your child's desired body weight. Multiply it by 3 if your child is sedentary, 5 if moderately active, 10 if very active.

3. Add the number from Step 1 (the number of calories your child needs to maintain bodily function) to the number from Step 2 (the number of calories your child needs to fuel activities).

> **C**hildren should remember that their fitness is in their hands. Make good decisions about what you eat and drink, when you exercise, when you sleep, not doing drugs. Don't get in the habit of letting life just happen— make good things happen.
>
> Karl Malone
> *professional basketball player*
> *(Utah Jazz)*

Teaching Your Child Food Cues

Now that you know the elements of a good diet and how it should be structured, the rest is easy. Right? Teaching your children to sit down daily to count calories and review nutrients is probably the last thing on your mind. I don't even have time (or the desire) to do it for myself! A simpler alternative is to use this information to help you and your child make healthy food choices.

▼ Eat a variety! No one food supplies everything you need. Not even a small group of foods can do the trick. Have a wide variety of healthful foods on hand to choose from. Try to sit down to meals that have representatives from the four food groups shown on the pyramid.

▼ Eat nothing in excess. Most nutritional or weight problems arise when you eat too much, even of a good thing.

▼ Homemade is best. While processed foods are certainly easier to prepare, they are not only more expensive than homemade meals, they also contain more fat, sodium, and sugars than you probably use in your cooking. And unless they are fortified, they probably contain fewer nutrients than fresh foods do. Teach your child how to prepare nutritious snacks like popcorn, celery and peanut butter, french bread pizza, and pretzels and cheese dip. Cook large quantities during meal preparation and then freeze some for another meal.

Guide children of various ages in different ways. For 2- to 5-year-olds, give foods fun names, such as spaghetti snakes or cauliflower snowballs. Get as much mileage out of Popeye eating spinach and Bugs Bunny eating carrots as you can. Assume your child will enjoy all foods; let your child's tastes develop without the bias of society. Involve the 6-to-11 set in cooking and shopping. Ask your child's opinion on which vegetables to buy or what to put in the salad (using options you can live with).

Set a good example by eating regular meals and making healthful food choices yourself. Act as a gatekeeper to control what foods come into the house. The most successful approach to raising a child with good eating habits is to let her control the amount of food she eats while you control the quality and type of foods she eats.

The Most Important Meal of the Day

You've heard it before, and the research supports it—your children will feel better if they eat breakfast. Breakfast gives the energy needed to stay awake in school as well as to fight the urge for an unhealthy snack later on. Ideally, the day's first meal should be the largest, with later meals proportionately smaller. The last meal of the day should be about 2 hours before bedtime.

America's number one choice for breakfast—cereal—can also be one of our healthiest meals as well. Cereal can be quick, easy, and rich in carbohydrates, calcium, fiber, and iron, plus low in fat. Make the most out of this meal by choosing the best cereals. Look for ones that are iron enriched and made from high-fiber bran. Avoid cereal with sugar added. Instead, put a sugar bowl on the table and let taste buds regulate. Also, avoid cereals that have lots of sodium or fat. If your child prefers sweetened cereals, jazz up a healthy one with fresh or dried fruit, nuts, raisins, or flavored yogurt and see if it turns his head.

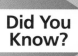
Did You Know?

Lucky Charms, Frosted Flakes, Honey Smacks, and Apple Jacks cereals average more than 6 to 8 teaspoons of sugar per bowl!

The Vegetarian Alternative

As more and more families are cutting back on their meat intake, the vegetarian alternative seems to be expanding. A vegetarian diet is usually low in fat and rich in carbohydrates, which makes it conducive to an active, healthy lifestyle. Yet the down side of vegetarianism is that animal products contain necessary nutrients, especially calcium and protein. You will need to plan ahead for your child to eat a vegetarian diet that includes all the needed nutrients.

Maintaining a well-balanced diet with vegetarian eating is not easy. Most doctors do not recommend vegetarian diets for young children, especially diets that cut out dairy products. Talk with a nutritionist if your family follows a vegetarian diet to be sure your child develops healthily. If your adolescent child chooses this route, you can read books together on vegetarian eating. Work with your child to develop sound, responsible eating habits.

Snacking Is a Fact of Life

As long as the sun shines and the rivers run, kids will be snackers. In fact, snacks contribute 30% or more of the calories in a teenager's diet. Depending on your child's activity level, a snack may be necessary to keep metabolism high and the brain in gear. Unfortunately, most foods consumed as snacks are high in fat, sodium, and simple sugars.

But snacking can be healthy. Plan ahead for snacks that fit into your family's nutritional scheme. Let your children have a snack before they get too ravenous and eat anything in sight. Snacking and TV seem to go hand in hand. Set rules, such as never eating while watching TV or only snacking on nutritious foods like apples and carrots. Encourage healthy snacks by keeping nutritious alternatives on hand. I keep fresh fruits, graham crackers, and yogurt at "kid accessible" levels in my kitchen to make it easy for my children to grab a healthy snack anytime. Our treats are squirreled away in areas only I have access to.

Tasty snacks that are rich in carbohydrates fuel muscles. Here are good foods to choose from.

Apples	Frozen fruit bars	Potatoes (baked)
Apricots	Frozen yogurt (lowfat)	Pretzels
Bagels	Gingersnaps	Raisins
Bananas	Grapes	Raw veggies
Breads	Melons	Rice cakes
Cereals	Oranges	Vanilla wafers
Crackers	Peaches	Yogurt (lowfat)
Fig bars	Pears	

Eating Out

The biggest growth in new restaurants today is in the "family restaurant" arena. That may sound like good news for us with kids, but it's not always so good if you're trying to eat healthfully. Burgers, fries, fried chicken, and meaty subs are staples in these venues. But you don't have to give up good eating habits while dining out. Help your child make good food choices.

In general encourage broth-based rather than cream-style soups. Load up at salad bars with lots of greens, raw veggies, and fruits (but limit high-fat salad toppings like cheese, eggs, and bacon bits, and go easy on the dressing). Order entrees described as steamed, boiled, broiled, poached, grilled, baked, or cooked in their own juices. Avoid those described as fried, crispy, breaded, scampi-style, creamed, buttery, au gratin, or served with gravy.

Although many fast food meals are high in fat and low in calcium and vitamins A and C, most restaurants now have foods that fit a healthy game plan. For breakfast select pancakes or eggs. Avoid breakfast sandwiches, which are often high in calories and fat. Instead of french fries, try a baked potato or a side salad. Grilled chicken is the best sandwich pick. Breaded chicken or fish is no better (and sometimes worse) than a hamburger. And when choosing a fast food sandwich, order it plain so you can control the condiments.

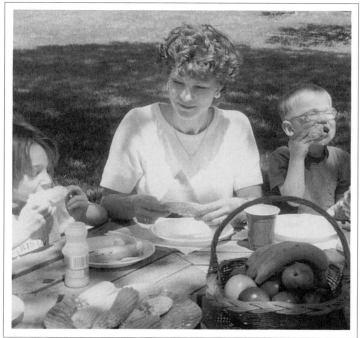

© Doug Brown

Did You Know?

To burn off one McDonald's Big Mac, large fries, and a milk shake would require a little over 2 hours of swimming, close to 3 hours of running, about 3-1/2 hours of aerobics, or almost 11 hours of golf!

Maintaining Healthy Weight

The key to healthy weight is maintaining low body fat and strong muscles. The best way to do this is to eat a lowfat diet *and* to stay active to burn calories. Studies have looked at people who just cut the fat in their diets, those who just did exercise, and those who did both. Researchers found that you'll take it off and keep it off easiest if you cut the fat and increase exercise.

Dieting doesn't mean introducing your child to a hard-core calorie-restricted regimen. Instead, focus on fats. Fats have twice the calories of proteins and carbohydrates. Excess dietary fat is also easily stored as body fat, whereas only a very small percentage of excess carbohydrate can be stored that way. Many people can eat as many fruits, vegetables, pastas, and grains as they like if they watch the amount of fat they consume.

Obesity Is a Problem

Obesity, which doctors define as anything from being mildly to severely overweight, affects as many as two in five American children, and the problem is getting worse. Between 1963 and 1980 obesity increased 54% among 6- to 11-year-olds, and 39% among 12- to 18-year-olds. And it's getting worse.

Because children have irregular growth spurts and body types, it is difficult to say when a child starts gaining too much weight. Nonetheless, addressing the issue in childhood gives a child the best chance of overcoming long-term problems.

Overweight teenage boys are twice as likely to die early as lean boys. And overweight teenagers of both sexes have a higher risk of serious disease before age 73, regardless of their weight in middle age. Teens in the top 25% in weight for their age are twice as likely to be diagnosed with coronary heart disease, seven times more likely to develop atherosclerosis, and nearly three times more likely to have gout by age 73 than their leaner peers.

Obesity is more than a physical problem in children. Society labels fat kids as lazy, sloppy, and lacking in self-control. In childhood kids develop their first self-impressions and their ideas of how they fit into the world. Of all the reasons children get teased, obesity is at the top of the list. Weight problems damage self-esteem and make it difficult for children to form friendships. In studies where they were asked to choose playmates, children as young as 5 and 6 ranked their overweight peers at the bottom of the list.

Because overweight parents often have overweight children, some people think that obesity is genetic. The facts in this area are not clear, but most seem to indicate that obese parents are more likely to pass on poor eating habits to their children than they are to pass on a "fat" gene. The gene that has been making headlines only controls how full you feel when eating, not what you put in your mouth. Likewise, some people believe that an unalterable "set point" controls body composition. In fact, sustained exercise programs may lower set points.

Advise your doctor of your child's weight loss goals. Most health professionals do not recommend that a child focus on a calorie-reduction diet. Quick losses often result in quick regains. Help your child focus instead on a lowfat diet. Lowfat diets, by nature, are low in calories. You want to help your child learn to make healthy eating choices that he can live with— for life. Making this a painless process means using no draconian methods.

> **K**eeping disciplined is one of my toughest obstacles in my quest for fitness, but watching the fat slip away and muscle developing gives me a great sense of accomplishment.
>
> Michelle Wright
> *country singer*

Do-It-Yourself Family Weight Loss Plan

A strong family support system is key to a child's mental health. If your child could stand to lose a little weight, your whole family should come together to support the effort. Don't worry—I'm not saying everyone has to eat 1,000 calories and three grapefruit a day. Most of the popular or trendy weight loss plans don't work well over time. Why? They aren't diets you can live with. If a weight loss plan isn't realistic over the long haul, it ain't gonna work. Instead, have your entire family focus on good eating.

Everyone will benefit, and everyone can be a winner. Here are some key points to make your diet a success.

- Eat every meal. Breakfast should account for at least a third of your child's daily calories, with the remainder spread throughout the day in meals and snacks.

- Include some favorite foods. Being deprived of every favorite just makes life difficult and dieters unhappy. Include regular small portions of whatever is your child's favorite, but look for the healthiest version of that subgroup—fig bars for cookies, gummi bears for candy, or lowfat frozen yogurt for ice cream, for example. If you offer small amounts of treats, often your child will be more eager to make this new eating plan work.

- Remember that nutritious eating can be rewarding. Children may revert to unhealthy eating habits because they get bored, the results of dieting aren't quick enough, they haven't found good alternatives to bad eating habits, or they don't have the necessary self-discipline. Be prepared for potential problems, and combat them with solutions. Give rewards. Set small goals. Keep trying new foods and recipes. Talk to your child about her feelings during this time, and help her work through them.

- Combine good eating habits with activity! While a lowfat diet can help your child drop excess fat, regular exercise helps keep the fat off.

- Be compassionate and empathic with your child during this time. Contrary to popular belief, obesity is not necessarily caused by a lack of personal courage or willpower. Just as you would tutor your child to improve his reading skills, give guidance and support for developing good eating habits, too.

Underweight Children and Eating Disorders

Although obesity is a problem for many youngsters, weighing too little can also be a problem. Young athletes, especially those involved in gymnastics, long-distance running, ballet, and wrestling, tend to focus on weight. More and more children are restricting their food intake because they are overly concerned about body weight. In a recent study of children ages 3 to 6 from Cincinnati, Ohio, nearly half of the children wanted to be thinner, and more than a third said they had tried to lose weight.

A person with anorexia nervosa has such an overwhelming desire to lose weight that she or he is willing to literally starve. Bulimia is a second eating disorder, characterized by bingeing on food and purging afterward. Both conditions are more common among teenage girls than boys. And they can be deadly, or leave lifelong physical and emotional scars. If you notice your child is getting thinner, whether you see her eating good meals or not, talk about it. If your child says his coach told him to lose weight, check with the coach. If the coach feels it's necessary, talk to your pediatrician. Have your child's body fat measured to be sure weight loss is advisable for health, and then make a long-term plan.

Don't go it alone if you think your child may have an eating disorder. There are mental as well as physical implications to this problem. Ask your pediatrician for guidance.

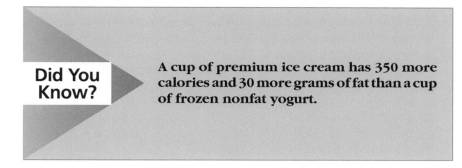

Did You Know? A cup of premium ice cream has 350 more calories and 30 more grams of fat than a cup of frozen nonfat yogurt.

Feeding a Young Athlete

A diet rich in complex carbohydrates, such as pasta, fruit, vegetables, and cereals, is important for every child. For an athletic child, however, a high-carb diet is even more important. Carbohydrates, in the form of glycogen, are stored in the muscles and provide fuel for sports. A high-carbohydrate diet will give your child the energy she needs to stay active.

Especially before and after competition, the best foods for your child are—you got it—carbohydrates! They are easy to digest and will fuel your child's muscles the quickest. Avoid fatty foods, which take longer to digest. Within an hour before exercise, avoid sugary foods. Sugar gives a temporary energy boost, but it is always followed by a "sugar low" that leaves your child more tired than normal.

Liquid foods leave the stomach faster than solids. So if you're short on time, your child can drink a fruit and yogurt shake, or a carbohydrate replacement drink (found in sporting goods stores).

Fluids are critically important for the active child. Dehydration is life threatening. Make sure your child drinks six to eight glasses of fluids a day. When it's hot and your child is active, he should drink 4 to 8 ounces of cool water every 15 minutes during activity. However, if your child says he feels bloated or waterlogged, he should stop. The actual amount of water needed depends on body size and the degree of sweating. Subtle signs of dehydration include dry eyes, nose, or mouth. Less subtle signs include absence of sweating, dizziness, and fatigue.

Sports drinks are useful if your child will be exercising more than 45 minutes. Gradually introduce a sports drink to be sure your child's stomach can tolerate it. Never give your child an untested drink (or any new food, for that matter) the day of competition. Avoid drinks made from more than 10% fructose (the fruit sugar found in fruit juice and some sodas). These can cause nausea and diarrhea during exercise. Energy bars are useful if your child will be working out longer than an hour or to quickly refuel muscles with carbohydrates after a strenuous workout. Be sure your child drinks lots of water along with the solid energy bar to dissolve the bar in the stomach.

Your young athlete does not need additional salts or other electrolytes during competition. However, studies have found that sports drinks that contain sodium improve water and glucose (muscle fuel) absorption.

Finally, make sure your child gets enough calories during intensive training. But remind your child to reduce food intake when activity levels drop.

What's a Carbohydrate-Rich Diet?

Your active child is supposed to eat lots of carbohydrates. Here's what your menu could look like if you were really trying to load up your child before competition.

- Breakfast—whole-grain cereal (cold or hot) with sliced banana, skim milk, bagel, melon
- Snack—fruit yogurt with granola sprinkles
- Lunch—tuna salad sandwich on whole-wheat bread, gingersnaps, apple, raw carrots, skim milk
- Snack—unbuttered popcorn, juice
- Dinner—stir-fried vegetables and chicken on wild rice, green salad, skim milk, sherbet with berries

Timing Meals Before Competition

Providing the right fuel before competition will give your child his best chance to succeed. Always serve familiar foods before competition. Don't try anything new because you won't know how it will be digested or affect performance. See Table 4.5 for more detailed tips.

	Table 4.5	Timing Meals Before Competition
Event	**Time of day**	**What and when to eat**
Swim meet	Morning	Have a carbohydrate-rich dinner the night before. Drink lots of water throughout the evening and morning. Eat a light breakfast of toast or cereal 1 or 2 hours before the event.
Soccer game	Noon	Have a carbohydrate-rich dinner the night before. Drink lots of water throughout the evening and morning. Have cereal, toast, or pancakes for breakfast (avoid fat). Eat an energy bar before the game with water. Drink a sports drink during the game if active for more than 45 minutes.
Football game	Afternoon	Have a carbohydrate-rich dinner the night before. Drink lots of water throughout the evening and morning. Have a large breakfast of cereal, toast, or pancakes (avoid fat) and a light lunch of noodles or a sandwich. Or have a hefty carbohydrate-rich brunch midmorning and a small snack about an hour before game time.
Basketball game	Evening	Focus on carbohydrates all day long. As always, drink lots of water through-out the day. Have a light dinner (avoid fats) about 2 hours before the game. If there's no time for dinner, have a midafternoon snack and another about an hour before the game. Fruit, pop-corn, muffins, and an energy bar with water are good choices.

What your children eat has a great impact on their fitness and well-being. It will help them grow bigger and stronger, as well as help fight disease. And by teaching kids to make healthy food choices and acquire tastes for healthy foods, we parents are giving them tools for a healthy lifestyle in the future. In the next chapter we'll look at how fitness within the family setting enables children to begin establishing lifelong habits that will help them stay active.

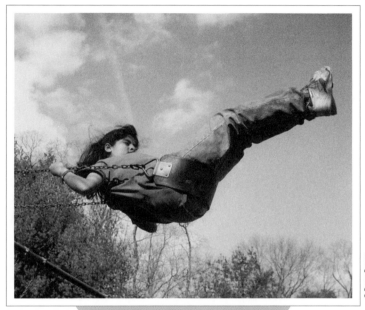

© Doug Brown

Fitness Is a Family Affair

Choose the activity that doesn't belong: taking out the trash; going for a walk; doing your taxes; visiting the dentist.

Did you choose the walk? The others are all important tasks that must be done regularly but are far from what anyone would call fun. On the other hand, going for a walk is an example of a fun fitness activity, which you should also do regularly. One of the many great things about fitness is that it need not be a chore or a necessary evil (like taxes and the trash). You or your child may think it nearly impossible to develop an active lifestyle, but it's not so hard as you may think. Research shows that within 3 weeks a new activity becomes habit—suddenly it's not so hard to do.

Activity Is Key

Being active is the key to improving endurance, strength, flexibility, and body composition. You already have two factors on your side in helping your child become more fit. First, a child's natural inclination is to be active. Sedentary kids are inactive because they've picked up cues from the world around them.

Second, your child will follow your lead. No one holds a greater influence over your child than you. She picks up your cues, spoken and unspoken, in all areas—including fitness. I often used to find myself

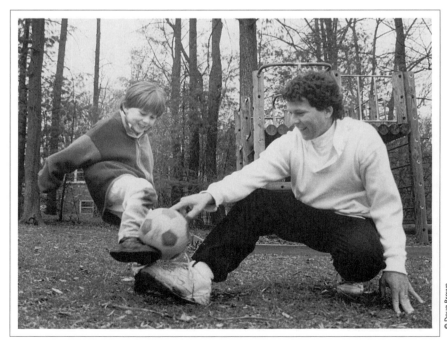

© Doug Brown

looking for the closest parking spot at the mall. The time I wasted driving around! It would have been quicker to just walk, and healthier too. But in retrospect, what frustrates me more is knowing that the message I sent my kids wasn't a healthy one. Beware: Your unspoken messages—what you do—make a more lasting impression than your words.

Supporting Your Child's Fitness Habit

Are you sending the right messages to your child? It's easy to say you want him to be active, but are you helping? Take this test and see.

Are You a Fitness Booster?

QUIZ Read each question and circle the answer that is the closest fit to your family situation. Tabulate your score at the end to see if you are a fitness booster.

1. Are you available for scheduled family fitness outings?
   a. always   b. sometimes
   c. never   d. We don't have fitness outings.

2. Do you remind your child to exercise at a particular time?
   a. yes   b. sometimes   c. no

3. Do you monitor your child's exercise progress?
   a. yes   b. sometimes   c. no

4. Do you exercise with your child?
   a. weekly   b. occasionally   c. I did once.   d. I never do.

5. Do you reward your child for a fitness activity well done?
   a. yes   b. sometimes   c. no

6. Do you monitor the amount of time your child watches TV?
   a. yes   b. sometimes   c. no

7. Do you take your child to the doctor for regular checkups or physicals?
   a. yes   b. sometimes   c. no

8. Do you keep healthy snacks in your home?
   a. yes   b. sometimes   c. no

9. Do you develop weekly menus to include a balance and variety of foods?

    a. yes　　　　　b. sometimes　　　　　c. no

10. Do you base your dinners around a meat dish?

    a. always　　　　　　　　b. 4 or 5 times a week
    c. 2 or 3 times a week　　d. rarely

11. If your child is over 12 years old, do you discuss peer use of drugs and alcohol?

    a. yes　　b. I did once.　c. I never have.

12. If your child is over 12 years old, have you introduced the concept of safe sex?

    a. yes　　　　　b. I did once.　　　　　c. no

13. Do you make sure your child gets at least 8 to 9 hours of sleep each night?

    a. yes　　　　　b. occasionally　　　　　c. no

14. Do you encourage your child to participate in a sport?

    a. yes　　　　　b. no

15. Do you budget money to purchase fitness equipment (shoes, balls, etc.) for your child?

    a. yes　　　　　b. occasionally　　　　　c. no

16. Do you talk to your child about his team's progress or the progress she is making in her sport?

    a. yes　　　　　b. occasionally　　　　　c. no

17. Do you (or another significant adult) attend your child's sport events?

    a. regularly　　b. occasionally　　　　　c. rarely

18. Do you discuss what your child is learning in physical education class?

    a. yes　　　　　b. occasionally　　　　　c. no

✓Scoring

1. a. 10　　b. 5　　c. 0　　d. 0
2. a. 5　　b. 3　　c. 0
3. a. 5　　b. 3　　c. 0
4. a. 10　　b. 5　　c. 1　　d. 0
5. a. 5　　b. 3　　c. 0
6. a. 10　　b. 5　　c. 0

7.	a. 10	b. 5	c. 0
8.	a. 5	b. 3	c. 0
9.	a. 5	b. 3	c. 0
10.	a. 0	b. 3	c. 4	d. 5
11.	a. 5	b. 1	c. 0
12.	a. 5	b. 1	c. 0
13.	a. 5	b. 2	c. 0
14.	a. 3	b. 0	
15.	a. 3	b. 2	c. 0
16.	a. 5	b. 3	c. 0
17.	a. 5	b. 3	c. 0
18.	a. 5	b. 3	c. 0

✓Results

More than 94—You are a true fitness booster, helping your child develop lifelong skills to help stay active for many years.

75 to 94—You've got the right idea, but you can do more to help your child enjoy an active lifestyle.

50 to 74—You need to work much harder to be sure your child embraces an active lifestyle.

Under 50—Be careful, you may be raising a couch potato. Make the commitment today to help your child benefit from an active lifestyle.

The Messages You Send

Telling your child to be more active will be much more effective if you yourself are active. And it will be most effective if you actually include your child in your activity.

Children of active mothers are twice as likely to be active as children of inactive moms. Apparently, fathers have an even greater influence. Active dads are 3-1/2 times more likely to have active kids than sedentary dads. And if you and your spouse both enjoy sports, your children are almost 6 times as likely to exercise. No other factors are so strongly correlated!

The more you get involved, the better. How often parents exercise with children is directly related to how often they exercise themselves. Consistency communicates to children something about how much we value exercise. Exercising with our kids not only contributes to their immediate physical activity level but also to the likelihood that they'll make exercise a long-term habit.

> ## My parents, my brothers, and my sister were all very active in sports. It was always a way of life with my family.
>
> Mary Lou Retton
> *Olympic gymnast*

On average, moms spend about the same amount of time exercising with a son as with a daughter, about 45 times a year. Dads, on the other hand, spend a lot more time exercising with their sons (about 50 times a year) than with their daughters (35 times a year). See Figure 5.1 for other statistics.

Figure 5.1 How Often Do Parents Exercise With Their Children?

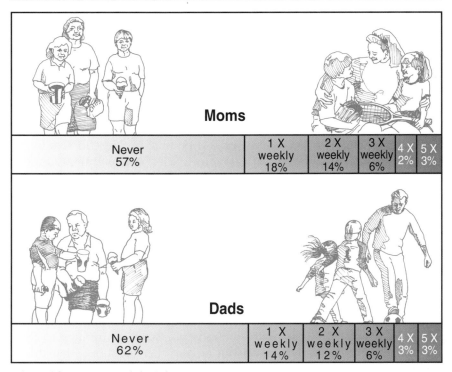

Moms

Never 57%	1 X weekly 18%	2 X weekly 14%	3 X weekly 6%	4 X 2%	5 X 3%

Dads

Never 62%	1 X weekly 14%	2 X weekly 12%	3 X weekly 6%	4 X 3%	5 X 3%

Adapted from Ross, et al. (1987).

Working out with your child can be a tough commitment when you must balance work, chores, and personal time. But the good news is that just as you are the greatest influence on your children, they can have a positive impact on your fitness level, too! While you're helping your kids become fit and healthy, they'll be doing the same for you.

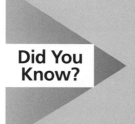

Did You Know?

In a recent study, parents were asked to rate their activity levels and those of their children. They perceived that the levels were fairly similar, but both estimates were actually too high. In reality, more than 70% of parents with children between the ages of 1 and 4 exercise moderately fewer than three times a week. More than 42% never exercise. And children generally mirror their parents.

Be a Positive Role Model

Your job, however, is a bit more complex than just working out with your child. You are his key motivator, cheerleader, teacher, enforcer, and friend.

So the pressure's on. Not only do you have to help your child choose to avoid drugs, alcohol, and sexually transmitted diseases, you're also responsible for her sweat factor! But don't worry. There are many ways to help your child develop a love of movement and activity, and they don't include your running a marathon. Here are the basics:

First, take care of yourself. When your child sees that you value your health and are willing to do things to preserve it, such as exercising regularly and eating a healthy diet, she will learn to respect her body and take care of it too.

Next, keep your eyes and your mind open to the wide array of activity possibilities. The road to fitness can take many turns. Remember that the health benefits of exercise come from activity—walking, running, biking, swimming, dancing, skipping, kicking, throwing, hiking, tumbling, to name just a few. One child's pleasure is another child's pain. Don't let your child give up on sports just because he can't throw a ball. Help him try a smorgasbord of activities to discover the ones he enjoys.

Finally, know you're being watched. Be a good sport. Follow sensible training techniques. If you exercise even though you're in pain, your child might too. If you are a poor loser, your child may become one. Act in a way you would want your child to emulate . . . because you *will* be imitated. Have you ever seen a parent pitch a fit at a softball game?

Chances are that person's son or daughter is doing the same thing at practice.

Whether we like it or not, we are similar to our parents in many ways. Be sure the messages you send your children are ones you will be proud of later in life. Review the messages listed in Table 5.1 and compare them to your own.

Table 5.1 What Messages Do You Send?	
Healthy messages	Unhealthy messages
• Exercising at least 3 times a week • Walking reasonable distances rather than driving (weather permitting) • Watching less and doing more! • Actively playing with your child • Getting enough sleep • Having fun when you exercise • Eating nutritionally balanced meals • Eating fruit or pretzels instead of cakes or candy bars as snacks	• Always using leisure time as sedentary time • Eating junk food or having a high-fat diet • Not attempting to regulate your body composition • Smoking, or drinking more than a little alcohol • Exercising irregularly—and moaning and groaning when you do • Saying you're too busy to exercise • Not exercising with your child

Real-Life Fit Families

The most successful families incorporate healthy living into all aspects of life. It won't work if you segment your "healthy living" to a specific time or day. Look for ways to develop family traditions that are active. My good friends the Wisor family came up with workable alternatives to sedentary living.

"I noticed my girls plopped in front of the TV as soon as they came home from school," Julie Wisor, mother of two, told me. "So our new rule is for every hour of TV we watch a day, we will also do something active. On days Kristin has gymnastics, that's not hard, but Katie has to plan ahead."

The Wisors also developed active family traditions, such as going for walks after dinner on Sundays and bringing a picnic of healthy foods for the whole family to cheer for Gary at softball games.

"We found we were becoming couch potatoes even on vacations—just going to the beach, eating, sunbathing, and eating some more. Now we plan at least one active holiday a year." Like the Wisors, you can go camping, hiking, or biking on your vacations. You can even train together for your trip.

As your children grow, involve them in exercise programs at home. "When Katie was little, she'd dance while I did my aerobics tape. Later, we'd go for walks or bike rides together," said Julie. By staying involved as your child progresses, as the Wisor's have, you will develop many sports to share by the time your child is in high school.

It is also important to balance an active schedule with down time. "Between work, church, and our sports activities, I felt we were being pulled in every direction," Julie said. "It seemed like we all were getting stressed out. Now we try to plan quiet time so we can relax, read, or just think."

Be sure your child gets enough sleep. Eight hours of sleep nightly is the average, but some children require more, while others need less.

Another important aspect of fitness is prevention. Take your child for regular medical checkups, including visits to a pediatrician, dentist, and optometrist. Be sure your child's vaccinations stay up-to-date, and keep tabs on where your medical records are.

Fitness Is Child's Play

Family fitness isn't quite as easy as one, two, three. It requires planning. But we can go a long way toward ensuring that our children will have an active life. How? As I said earlier, begin by being active and exercising with our kids. We encourage them through our words and actions. We praise their efforts and go to their games. We can ask them to show off their skills.

Make sure fitness is available to your child. Be aware of what the school and community have to offer. Help find friends to work out and play with. If your schedule won't allow you to take your child to various sporting events or practices, enlist family or friends. Perhaps you can trade rides with a neighbor. Or contact an organization such as Big Brother/Big Sister to help get support for your child's activities when you can't be there.

Don't allow bad habits to start. Monitor your child's television time. Help your child develop a schedule that includes time for meals, active recreation, homework, TV, and reading. Be firm about enforcing good habits. Here are three goals to work for:

1. Make sure your children have an abundance of opportunities for enjoyable and vigorous activities suited to their developmental ages.

2. Help children develop basic skills and interests so that they can participate in a variety of activities that suit their interests and abilities.

3. Give children the confidence to continue trying to improve their fitness level and reach their fitness potential.

What Motivates Children?

One reason parents are so influential to children's interest in sports is that most parents who exercise enjoy doing so. Children see their parents having fun and want to join in. As we all know, a child's number one interest is having fun. Be aware of what motivates children to exercise (see Table 5.2). Take steps to encourage your child to embrace an active lifestyle. Learn what cues work for your child.

Table 5.2 Fitness Turn-Ons and Turn-Offs	
What turns kids on to fitness	**What turns kids away from fitness**
• Having fun • Feeling successful • Playing with peers • Sharing experiences with family • Experiencing a variety of activities • Having an enthusiastic coach or teacher • Feeling that an active lifestyle is their own choice	• Putting winning above all else • Never improving • Getting injured too often • Feeling forced to play through pain • Doing the same thing over and over • Getting ridiculed by friends, family, or coach • Not having a say in the sports they play

Reprinted from American Footwear Association.

Did You Know? Although 45% of children age 10 play team sports outside of school, that number drops to 26% by the end of high school.

Children stick with a sport because they have fun. Aside from your duty as a good role model, be a good coach and cheerleader. Be sure your child is having fun in sports and do your best to keep fun the major factor in your child's exercise experience. Here are some dos and don'ts for family fitness:

Dos

▼ Listen to your child when she talks about sports. Look for what motivates her and what dampens her spirit. Focus on what pleases your child, not what pleases you.

▼ Develop an understanding of what your child wants from sports— not all children want the same thing. Some children want to be part of a team, others want a challenge, while others want to be able to shout a lot. Help your child pick a sport that meets his needs.

▼ Recognize your child's needs and a find a balance between your needs and hers. As important as activity is for kids, make sure it's in perspective and in sync with the whole family.

▼ Keep your perspective. Don't expect a child to be able to keep up with you. Also remember that each child is different, and don't judge your child by what your neighbor's child can do.

▼ Plan activities that are fun, improve skills, and lead to self-knowledge. These are the motivation for kids who stick to sports.

▼ Ask positive questions after your child participates in sports: "What do you enjoy most?" or "What did you learn?" Ask about a specific skill you know your child is trying to enhance or is proud of. Focusing on these areas will help children continue to enjoy sports, whether or not they're on a winning team.

▼ Help your child develop a good base of strength, endurance, and flexibility. These basics are the stepping stones to all sports.

▼ Allow your child to be active in developing his own fitness program. Gradually allow him to become more and more independent in pursuing it.

▼ Reward the process of fitness rather than the final outcome. Being a player, getting in shape, having fun—these should be the goals. If, along the way, your child becomes a state champion, all the better.

> **F**ind sports that the family can do together, but don't live your past sports goals through your children. Encourage and participate, but remember to let children be children.
>
> *Karl Malone*
> *professional basketball player*
> *(Utah Jazz)*

Don'ts

▼ Don't force kids into participating. Provide options and assistance in helping your child choose a sport or workout. Don't try to live out your childhood dreams in your son's or daughter's activities.

▼ Don't berate or belittle your child. Mistakes happen. Winning isn't everything. Fun is.

▼ Sports should not be torture. Monitor practice, training, and games.

▼ Don't act like exercise is drudgery or good nutrition tastes bad. Project fitness and a good diet as interesting and enjoyable.

Fun Family Activities

Developing a family fitness program requires you to take into account the abilities and interests of everyone in your family. Marathoners can't really take their children on long runs, nor would a child fit into an adult softball league. But there are numerous ways you can exercise and play sports with your child.

Play With Me

I tried to teach my child with books;
He gave me only puzzled looks.
I tried to teach my child with words;
They passed him by, oft unheard.
Despairingly I turned aside,
"How shall I teach this child?" I cried.
Into my hands he put the key.
"Come," he said, "play with me."

—Author unknown

Reprinted from Teaching Elementary Physical Education (January 1993).

Fitness Activities

Children who see their parents regularly exercising will want to join in. But your child can't necessarily train as intensely or as long as you do. How can you work out together?

Aerobics

Invite your child to dance with you. Encourage him to move with the music, but don't force him to follow the routine exactly if he doesn't want to. If the routine is too hard, encourage him to hold his arms lower, or not to jump and step as much as you do. If the workout is broken into sections, such as warm-up, aerobic, strengthening/toning, and stretching, your child may want to do just one section with you. Children over age 8 should be able to increase their fitness level to enjoy the aerobic and calisthenic aspects. There are also numerous children's exercise tapes available that can give a parent a good workout too.

Bicycling

Bicycling is a great family activity. A toddler can ride in a child's seat on your bike, but as your child gets older she can ride beside you. A small child riding a tricycle or a very small two-wheeler pedals doubly fast to keep up with you, so it's not a good idea to take her on long rides at that age. But a child age 10 and up can handle half-day rides with ease. Everyone in the family should wear a helmet.

Canoeing

Children ages 10 and up enjoy family canoe trips. Be sure to put your child in the front of the canoe, so that the bulk of the paddling is done and supervised by the parent in the back.

Hiking/Backpacking

Just like walking, hiking is a great way to exercise with your family. Adjust the pace so that the slowest family member is comfortable. If the adult is carrying a heavy pack, an unencumbered child can typically keep up along a moderate trail. Even a toddler can join in the fun, sitting in a pack on a parent's back.

Jumping Rope

Many adults overlook the aerobic benefits of jumping rope. It's hard work, it strengthens your heart and lungs, and it's fun! This is one sport the whole family can participate in, and in many cases, your child will be delighted to teach you the ropes.

Martial Arts

Your child can develop strength, flexibility, self-esteem, and discipline from a variety of martial arts. You can, too. Classes often include people of different ages and sexes; the whole family can progress together and reap the benefits.

Running

Running is a great lifelong exercise, but due to the various speeds and distances involved, it is not usually a good sport to do with a child. If you enjoy running and want to involve your child, be sure to run a step behind so you never encourage her to go farther or faster than she is able. You can also take your child to a track and let her go at her own pace. You'll be able to keep an eye on her while you work out. When she tires, have her play or read in the field inside the oval.

Skating

In-line skating, roller skating, and ice skating are all great activities that can be enjoyed at any age. Be sure you child wears appropriate padding to reduce injuries, and do not encourage high-speed skating until he is comfortable with stopping and turning. If you use wheeled skates, outings along exercise trails are great for the whole family, but circular arenas are better when skating with young children.

Skiing

If your child can walk, he can probably learn to ski. And no one is really too old to learn. Whether it's water or snow skiing, your whole family can get a great workout. Due to the endurance needed for cross-country skiing, adults and children often do not keep a similar pace over the long haul (just like with running), and thus it's not generally a good family fitness activity, unless the children are older or the parents are willing to carry toddlers in a backpack.

Swimming

Many children learn to swim at a young age. But fitness, or lap, swimming rarely holds their interest because they can't talk or look at the scenery as they work out. You may want to take your school-age children to a pool with a lifeguard on duty when you do laps and let them play as you swim. Seeing you working out sends a good message. You can even encourage them to do a few laps, but don't let it become drudgery. Try games like Marco Polo or Toss the Stone, or develop relay races.

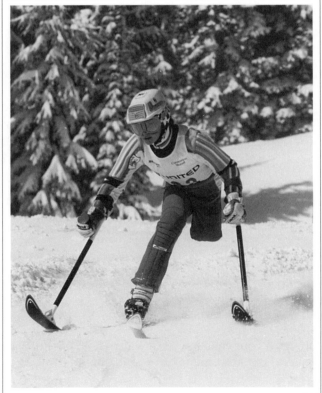

© Bruce Barthel. Courtesy of Disabled Sports USA.

Tag/Hide and Seek

Many childhood games can get your blood going. Tag encourages a love of running and activity. And while hiding doesn't require much work, chasing back to home will get you sweating. When playing with children, give them a handicap to make the game competitive for all. But don't be too obvious about the handicap—it can be demeaning.

Walking

Children over age 6 should be able to keep up with you on an easy walk. Together you can gradually go longer so that your child is walking briskly for 20 to 30 minutes. Even a toddler can join in the fun, sitting in a pack on a parent's back or being pushed in a stroller. Keep the conversation lively, talking about nature, life, friends, and future vacations and dreams.

Weights and Exercise Machines

Rowers, bicycles, steppers, and cross-country ski machines provide a good workout, but most aren't made for children to use. Not only do they not fit a child's body, *they also can be dangerous.* Children have lost fingers and broken bones putting hands in places they were not meant to go. Unless the machine was made for children, don't let your child use or play around your exercise machine.

> Always make getting fit fun with a wide variety of activities. Challenge your children to participate and reward them when they do well. Never, ever push them too hard or belittle their efforts. Always stress positive feedback.
>
> Steve Wright
> *professional football player*
> *(LA Raiders)*

Sports

Playing sports with your child is a great way to help her improve her skills as well as learn about sportsmanship and teamwork. But remember that no one ever enjoyed playing with bossy kids. So don't get too bossy playing with your child. It's usually best not to compete with your child; rather, use this time to have fun, teach your child through example, and get an easy workout. See Table 5.3 for some reasons that kids play sports—and reasons that they drop out.

Table 5.3 Why Kids Stay Active	
Why kids like to play sports	**Why kids drop out of sports**
• **To have fun** • **To improve their skills** • **To stay in shape** • **To do something they're good at** • **Because competing with peers is fun**	• **Practice isn't fun!** • **They find sports to conflict with academic demands.** • **They don't get to play or be active enough.** • **They miss out on social occasions because of sports.** • **They don't get help improving their skills.** • **Too much emphasis is placed on winning.**

Reprinted from American Footwear Association.

If your child's goal is to improve skills, help out, but approach it cautiously. Although I've had great relationships with many coaches and teachers, I've also enjoyed going home and having time to myself. If your parent-child relationship turns into a coach-child relationship, neither of you will have down time or a chance to cool out. If your child wants to seriously work on improving his sports skills more than can be accomplished through low-key workouts with you, then get a coach or sign him up for a class or league. Your child will always benefit from playing with you, but your time together should be fun. Many parents enjoy playing these sports with their children. Our sport selection chart (Table 5.4) provides assessments to help you make the right choices for your family.

Table 5.4 Choose a Sport That Fits Your Family Lifestyle

Sport	Goal			
	Endurance	Strength	Flexibility	Motor control
Aerobic dance	G	A	A	A
Backpacking	G	A	P	P
Baseball/softball	P	A	A	A
Basketball	A	A	P	G
Bowling	P	P	A	A
Cross-country skiing	G	A	A	H
Cycling	G	A	P	A
Field hockey	A	P	P	G
Football (touch)	P	A	P	A
Golf	P	P	A	A
Gymnastics	P	G	G	G
Handball/racquetball	A	P	P	G
Hockey	A	P	P	G
Horseback riding	P	A	P	A
Lacrosse	G	A	P	G
Martial arts	A	A	G	G
Ping Pong	P	P	P	G
Rope skipping	G	A	P	G
Rowing/canoeing	G	A	P	A
Running	G	A	P	P
Skating	G	P	P	A
Skiing (downhill)	P	P	P	A
Soccer	G	A	P	G
Swimming	G	A	P	P
Tennis/badminton	A	A	P	G
Track and field	G	A	A	A
Volleyball	P	P	P	G
Walking/hiking	G	P	P	P
Weight training	P	G	P	A
Wrestling	P	G	G	A

Legend
G = This is a good choice to reach your goal.
A = This sport is an adequate choice to reach your goal.
P = This sport is a poor choice to reach your goal.
L = Cost is relatively low for this sport.

			Cost		
Health	Family-friendly	Minimum age	Time	Money	Competitive?
G	G	3	L	L	N
G	G	10	H	H	N
A	A	5	M	M	Y
G	P	7	M	M	Y
A	G	6	M	M	Y
G	A	9	M	H	N
G	G	8	L	M	N
G	P	8	H	M	Y
A	A	7	M	H	Y
A	A	10	M	H	Y
A	P	3	M	H	Y
A	P	10	M	H	Y
G	P	10	H	H	Y
A	G	10	M	H	Y
G	P	10	H	H	Y
A	G	4	L	M	N
P	G	6	L	L	Y
G	G	4	L	L	N
G	A	8	H	M	N
G	A	5	L	L	N
G	A	8	L	M	N
A	G	8	H	H	N
G	P	6	H	M	Y
G	G	3	M	M	Y
A	P	8	M/L	M	Y
G	A	5	M	L	Y
A	A	10	M	M	Y
G	G	3	L/M	L	N
A	A	8	L	L	N
P	A	5	M	L	Y

M = Cost is relatively moderate for this sport.
H = Cost is relatively high for this sport.
Y = This is usually a competitive sport.
N = This is usually an uncompetitive sport.

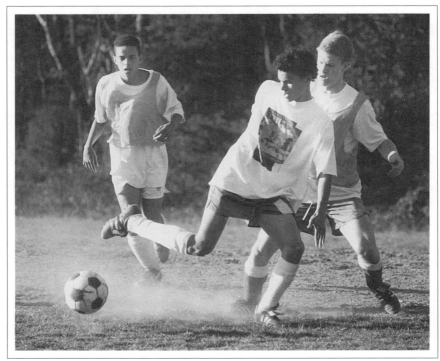

© Doug Brown

Golf

Golf is a lifelong sport that can be enjoyed at any age. Take your toddler to play miniature golf. Children under age 12 can learn a lot and enjoy three-par courses or pitch-and-putts.

Soccer, Basketball, Football, Hockey, Softball, and Baseball

You can begin to teach your young child skills that she can use in a variety of sports. Ball handling, running, sprinting, skating, and shooting are important skills that a parent and child can practice together. You can even enjoy drills using these skills. (Usually, however, the different skill levels between parent and child mean that competitive games aren't wise until the child reaches her mid-teens.)

Tennis and Racquetball

Children as young as 5 years old can begin tennis and learn to keep up an easy rally within a year. Doubles are a great family activity; pair two children against one adult or an adult and child against an adult to keep the game fun. Allow your child to modify his serve if necessary.

The more active you get with your child, the more rewarding your own fitness pursuits will be. And you'll have a front row seat for watching your child develop into a vigorous, well-rounded adult. The next chapter will focus on how school can help children learn about lifelong skills that will help them stay active.

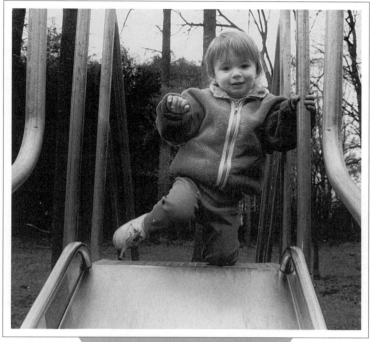

© Doug Brown

6

Getting Fit
in School

What was your school physical education experience like? I remember ugly, smelly uniforms that nearly stood up by themselves by the end of the week. We seemed to stand around in lines for hours in a drafty multipurpose room, waiting for a turn in the limelight. I still cringe when I think about the team captains choosing up sides. My health education began and ended with personal hygiene.

For many, physical education was nothing more than organized recess. The name was a misnomer: There wasn't much that was physical about it, and it wasn't very educational. Let's hope your child's experience is better. The time spent in physical education and the quality of instruction vary from state to state and from school to school. Physical education at its best has great benefits for kids, both short-term and long-term.

What Kids Should Learn in Physical Education

"Those who can, do. Those who can't, teach. And those who can't teach, teach PE." This old joke speaks volumes about the value our culture places on physical education. It is often the first subject cut when budgets need to be trimmed. Many school board members assume physical education is fun and games, with no intrinsic value. In fact, there are a number of important benefits to good physical education, and many don't have anything to do with sweat!

Physical education is an ideal place for children to learn the value of being active, the rewards of teamwork, and the nobility of fair play. Physical educators have great opportunities to debunk myths about physical activity, such as the need to have highly developed sports skills to be active or to exercise vigorously to get any benefits.

Many of the skills your child learns in physical education can be carried over into other aspects of life: self-discipline, goal setting, self-esteem and confidence, and teamwork.

Sports helped keep me motivated to stay in school. I enjoyed the teamwork and working for a common goal.

Michelle Wright
country singer

Physical education also can be a great place for children to learn the relationships between exercise, diet, and health. Yet too many children (and adults) still see physical education merely as a class where jocks get good grades. You need to look past this and to value fitness education, even if your child isn't active in sports. A good physical *fitness* education teaches jocks and nonjocks the value of being active over a lifetime. Sadly, most children (even jocks) grow up to lead sedentary lifestyles. Of course, it doesn't have to be that way.

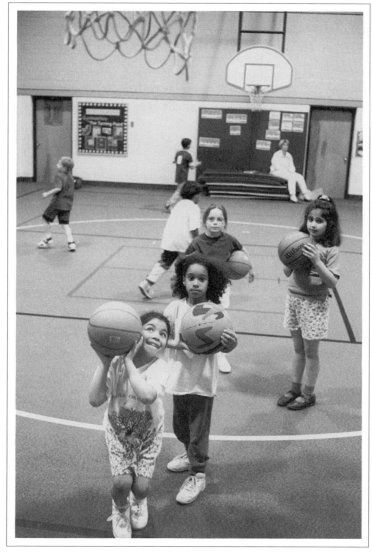

© Doug Brown

Status Quo Physical Education

Most parents are surprised at how little physical education their children receive. You might also be surprised at what is (and is not) being taught. Between changing clothes, getting instructions, and setting up lessons, on an average less than 9% of physical education class time is spent being vigorously active. For a child who takes 30 minutes of physical education, 3 times a week, that comes to about 8 minutes of exercise.

Many school programs still center on competitive sports, such as football and basketball, instead of lifetime sports, such as walking and aerobics. Participation in varsity sports should not replace physical education. In general, varsity athletes know no more (and often less) about maintaining healthy lifestyles. Grades based on skill levels discourage slow developers. Likewise, teachers who let children choose teams also put unfair pressure on the less physically gifted children. Children learn most when hearing, seeing, and doing. Good physical educators provide students with physical and mental challenges, not just lectures.

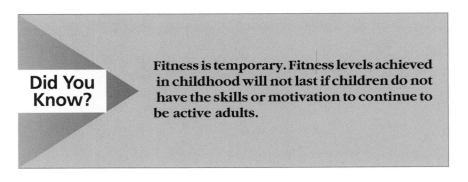

Did You Know?

Fitness is temporary. Fitness levels achieved in childhood will not last if children do not have the skills or motivation to continue to be active adults.

Quality Physical Education

Physical education is changing. Creative teachers are finding ways to make all children who try feel like winners. They focus on empowering children with skills to enjoy sports as well as improve fitness. What is a good program? The National Association for Sports and Physical Education (NASPE) has these suggestions:

▼ Physical education needs to take place daily. There is a positive correlation between physical fitness and a child's ability to concentrate and learn. Daily physical activity enhances book learning! Daily activity not only helps children develop regular fitness habits, it also helps them with their other lessons—daily.

▼ Physical education should be more than sweat. Your child should experience a smorgasbord of activities, should be taught skills that will allow him to excel in these activities, and should learn how to incorporate activity into his life's routine. What else should he learn? That activity plays a key role in health and well-being.

▼ Physical education should focus on the process, not the product. What's important is not how far a child can kick the ball, it's that she can kick a ball, enjoys doing it, and does it regularly. And that she can run, jump, and dance, too! All children who participate and improve their skills should be rewarded, not just those who are the most gifted. Physical education should accommodate the needs and developmental levels of all students, regardless of physical and mental ability.

▼ Physical education should be taught by certified physical education instructors. Children taught by trained professionals are more likely to perform better on fitness tests and have lower body fat than children taught by classroom instructors.

▼ Physical education should be progressive and fun. Your child's lifelong perception of fitness may be based on how he does in school physical education. If he has fun and improves, he will be more likely to stay active in adulthood. Physical education should be inclusive; everyone should play, and participation and improvement (not natural talent) should be rewarded.

▼ A child's fitness level should be monitored annually. Together children and teachers can develop goals based on fitness level. By setting realistic goals and attaining them, your child will feel like (and be) a winner!

> **O**rdinary people accomplish extraordinary things every day. In every case, they are ordinary people who dare to imagine an extraordinary triumph and then set out to attain what they have envisioned.
>
> Marilyn King
> *two-time Olympic pentathlete*

What You See Is What You Get

In many subjects, it's hard to tell what your child is learning. Math, science, and history aren't areas that noticeably affect the daily life of a child. But physical education is. In many schools, the traditional "drill sergeant" physical educator has been replaced by a fitness enthusiast who imparts a love of activity and healthful living to children. And it will show!

Physical education is practical knowledge about how to do better and live healthier. We know your children are learning if they are enthusiastic about sports, eager to try new skills, and conscious about the role diet and exercise play in their lives.

Does Your School Make the Grade?

QUIZ

This series of questions developed by nationally acclaimed physical educator Charles Kuntzleman, EdD, addresses your child's physical education program. Rate each question from 0 to 3, then total your responses.

- 1 means your school doesn't seem to address this area.
- 2 means your school addresses this area, but not very well.
- 3 means your school is doing a good job here.
- 0 means you don't know the answer (you get 0 points).

_____ 1. Our school physical education program has clearly defined and measurable goals and objectives, and the program is evaluated on the basis of these goals and objectives.

_____ 2. Our school sets aside at least 30 minutes a day for each child to exercise vigorously, regardless of physical ability.

_____ 3. Our school encourages extracurricular physical activity by helping parents find community-based leagues and classes or by coordinating school programs to complement after-school activities to be sure each child exercises daily.

_____ 4. Our school teaches not just how to exercise but also why exercise is important.

_____ 5. Our school regularly measures each child's strength, flexibility, and cardiovascular endurance and reports back to me areas where my child needs to improve.

_____ 6. Our school tracks and rewards my child's progress in these measurements.

_____ 7. Our school teaches lifetime activities (such as walking, aerobic dance, and strength training), not only competitive sports.

_____ 8. Our school's physical education program emphasizes fitness, basic skills, fun, and participation rather than skill development and competition.

_____ 9. My child's teachers (both physical educators and classroom instructors) look fit and project an active, healthy lifestyle.

_____ 10. My child enjoys physical education and looks forward to class.

_____ 11. My school offers lowfat lunches, including 2% milk, fresh fruits, vegetables, and legumes.

_____ 12. My school does not sell soft drinks, candy, or other nonnutritious foods during school hours.

✓Scoring

Add the total number of points.

✓Results

Over 26—You are one lucky parent! Your school system is outstanding and offers a well-rounded program for your child.

16 to 26—Your child's school is above average, but it needs help from you and other parents to really impact student fitness.

Under 16—Either you (how many zeros did you put down?) or your child's school isn't accepting responsibility for your child's fitness. Better get moving!

Reprinted from Kuntzleman (1991).

Health and Fitness Are Schoolwide Concerns

Just as healthy choices should be integrated into all components of your child's lifestyle, so should physical education be integrated in all aspects of a school and its curriculum. Classroom teachers and physical educators can coordinate efforts to be sure the fitness message is presented on all fronts.

Classroom teachers control recess and other free time that can be used for fitness-related activities. They can also integrate fitness concepts into classroom topics. For example, nutrition and body composition can be discussed in health and science; distance, time, and calorie measurements can be studied in math; and researching and writing about the role of exercise in lifestyle would be a great theme for English class.

The Exercise Across America challenge is a perfect example of how classroom teachers can work fitness into a variety of studies. This motivational activity challenges students to pick different U.S. states and to exercise their way across them. Each time a child exercises (by walking, biking, running, or doing another activity measured in distance), mileage accumulates until she reaches the goal distance for the state of her choice. Teachers have used this challenge to teach children about maps, compasses, heart rates, local history, and geography, all in the privacy of the schoolyard. For information about Exercise Across America, call 1-800-776-ARFA.

Creative Walking also offers great motivational and educational programs for classroom teachers. For information contact Creative Walking, PO Box 50296, Clayton, MO 63105, or call 314-721-3600. Another source of good ideas for classroom teachers is Fitness Finders, 133 Teft Rd., PO Box 160, Spring Arbor, MI 49283; phone 517-750-1500.

> **J**ust as science and math train the mind, a good physical education helps students develop and learn to use their bodies. Certainly, any concerned individual would not willingly give a child half an education.
>
> **Arnold Schwarzenegger**
> *actor and fitness advocate*

Be a Cafeteria Supporter

School lunch doesn't have to leave a bad taste in your child's mouth. I remember from my own childhood plates of unrecognizable and often inedible vegetables with mystery meats swimming in pools of grease. Today's school cafeterias, though, have foods that interest more children than ever before. But that doesn't mean the food is good for them.

If your child is like most, his school's lunch program is probably high in fat and sodium and low in fiber and other nutrients. Schools are caught between a rock and a hard place. They need to provide low-cost meals, they must prepare foods students will eat, and to save money they base meals on foods subsidized by the government (usually high-fat dairy products).

The government regulates the nutritional content of meals they subsidize. They promote calorie-dense foods because some youngsters from low-income areas get most of their nutrition through the school lunch. One stressed-out food-service provider told me that at times she has had to pour a teaspoon of oil over a meal to meet the government's requirement for fat! But things are changing.

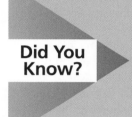

Did You Know?

A chemical analysis of lunches provided in one California elementary school found that they contained almost 10% more fat than meals normally recommend by health professionals.

In 1990 the Citizens Commission on School Nutrition issued a report recommending that lunches be limited to an average of 35% of calories from fat, with no more than a third of these from saturated fat. Fresh fruits, fresh vegetables, and legumes should be served much more frequently to increase students' consumption of fiber and vitamins. Meals should be low in salt, with no more than 1,000 milligrams of sodium per lunch. And, relatively nonnutritious foods that compete with school lunches, such as soft drinks, candy, and chips, should not be sold at school during school hours.

Implementing these recommendations is much easier said than done. Many parents have a hard time getting their kids to eat nutritious meals at home. What happens at school when you're not there to provide encouragement? Nutritious meals have to be packaged so that children will eat them.

Good school food-service directors have found ways to combine great nutrition with the appearance of those beloved fast foods. They add whole-wheat flour to pizza crust, install salad bars, and serve baked potatoes with lowfat toppings. They also reduce the fat in ethnic dishes, serving bean burritos and stir-fried chicken and vegetables. Plus they work with teachers and parents to teach students nutrition.

Successful programs get the whole school involved. Teachers can present nutrition education that directly relates to cafeteria offerings. Coaches and student leaders can promote lowfat, complex carbohydrates. But it's not easy.

To provide help in improving school lunch programs, the Public Voice for Food and Health Policy publishes *Serving Up Success*. For a copy send $15 to PV, 1101 14th St. SW, Suite 710, Washington, DC 20005, or call 202-371-1840.

The Competition Increases After School

With more parents working and crime invading once-safe neighborhoods, after-school pick-up games may become a thing of the past. Many schools are developing after-school programs with the primary goal of keeping kids safe. A secondary goal should be to get them fit.

A school with a limited daily physical education program can enhance its outreach by offering quality intramural programs after school. Intramurals are great for kids who enjoy sports but don't have the interest or skill to play on a varsity team. Team sports, such as volleyball, basketball, and softball, are the basics, but many schools are also developing aerobic dance programs, weight training and conditioning, and martial arts. If your school doesn't offer such programs, check with your local recreation department or church or community league.

Participation and sportsmanship should rule intramural programs. They should be voluntary and open to all students of all abilities. Children should be in charge of what is offered. Adults should be sure the programs are safe and fair.

But one problem with an intramural sports program, frankly, is that kids don't think it's cool. It's cool to play varsity sports; it's cool to hang out at the mall. But few children think it's cool to play intramurals. This perspective has to change. In part it is due to society's putting only elite athletes on pedestals. Student and athletic leaders need to develop plans to get students to try intramurals. Usually, once they get involved, they're hooked!

Be a Booster

Too often, people expect the school system to teach children everything from basic math and reading to computer programming, career development, and moral and ethical behavior—the list goes on. But that's not right or realistic. Your school should complement learning experiences you support at home. Parents can get involved by working with teachers. But their support is also crucial at school board meetings and at budget time.

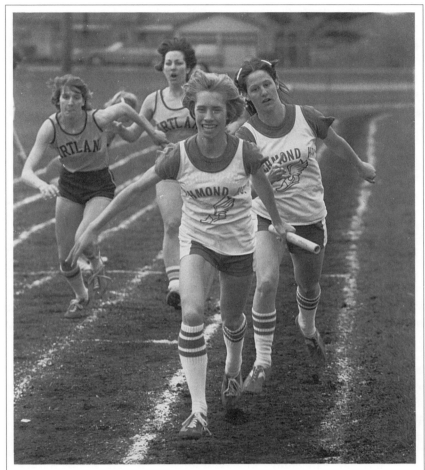

Courtesy of American Running and Fitness Assoc.

Help Out at Your Child's School

You can work with your child's teachers and schools to help not only your child but also the physical education program as well. Meet with your child's physical educator to determine what benchmarks are set for the coming year, and help your child in attaining them. You can also coordinate family fitness activities with those at school so that your child will get a well-rounded program. For example, if your child is playing soccer in class, why not take him to a college soccer game? Or if there will be a project on good nutrition, focus on healthy foods at home, too.

Can you volunteer? Many parents volunteer in the classroom, but you could volunteer on the playing field. Too often a single physical educator must supervise 40 children with various abilities over an entire playing field. This leads to lots of dead time, with children waiting for drills or games to be started. Having one more supervisor would reduce waiting and increase activity time. Other volunteer projects include getting free handouts for students, making copies of important information, organizing a fitness fair, and developing bulletin boards.

Did You Know?

It doesn't cost a lot to keep a school's athletic facilities open after school for community use. The biggest expense is for supervising the activities. Parents and community volunteers can work together to keep these great facilities open, safe, and used to their fullest.

Does your community have a sports-oriented doctor or another sports medicine professional? Why not ask that person to speak to your child's class about fitness, training, injury prevention, or healthy lifestyles.

Are you involved with a local fitness or sports club? See if your group can "adopt" a school or classroom. Your club may be able to share equipment, provide instructors, or do fund raising. What's more, nothing better motivates children than seeing important role models—*parents*—support fitness.

Think about your school's fitness facilities. Do they have a gym? A good playground? Equipment to play a variety of sports? Talk to the physical educator or other teachers to find out what is needed. You can develop a school booster club to help fund sports programs. Booster clubs not only help purchase needed equipment, they also support curriculum, teaching philosophies, and programs. For information on developing a booster club

Did You Know?

Your school's ability to teach your child is a local issue. The federal government provides little input or income. Almost all curriculum choices come down to parents' demands. Demand the best! And put your tax money where your mouth is. We'll all be paying a lot more in future health care costs if our children don't develop healthy lifestyles.

in your school, contact the Boosters Clubs of America, 200 Castlewood Dr., North Palm Beach, FL 33408; phone 407-842-4100. They can give you free information on how to raise money, mobilize support, and get things done.

Lobby for Good Physical Education

Too often the only people advocating physical education in the schools are the physical educators—and their quest looks a little too self-serving to convert people who do not understand the importance of the subject. Be an advocate for quality physical education.

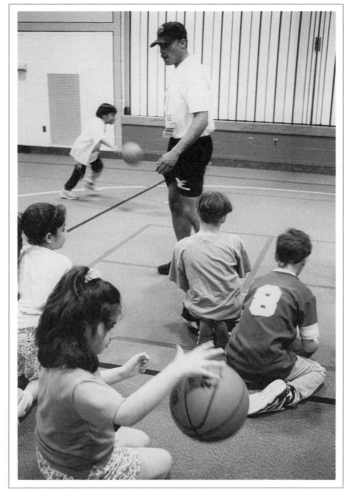

© Doug Brown

Most governmental bodies are looking for ways to cut budgets. Help your schools cut the fat while keeping the meat. Many schools have eliminated physical educators and put the responsibility of physical education on classroom teachers. Has that happened in your district? Perhaps your school can send classroom teachers to workshops to enhance their physical education skills. Or maybe your school could hire one physical educator (or consultant) to develop curriculum or lesson plans for classroom teachers.

If you think your school's physical education department isn't up to snuff, contact your state's Department of Education and ask about state physical education requirements. Is your school living up to the standards?

Remember, the squeaky wheel gets the oil. Let school board members, parents, school administrators, and other policymakers know the importance of physical education. Give them facts and figures on how to improve it. For information to help make the physical education program at your school the best it can be, contact the National Association for Sports and Physical Education, 1900 Association Dr., Reston, VA 22091; phone 703-476-3410. Ask for their "SPEAK" kit.

Schools can't be expected to cure all of society's ills. But schools are one system that almost all American children go through, and they can make an enormous impact. Help your school improve the health and fitness of our children. Your school and community hold a wealth of fitness opportunities. Next I'll discuss how you can access community-based programs.

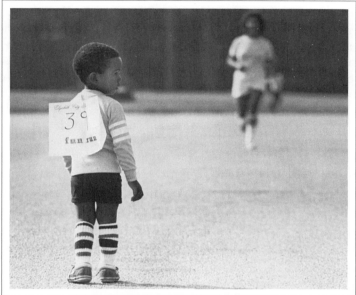

Community
Fitness and
Sports Programs

More than 20 million children in America play sports in community programs, such as those offered through YMCAs and YWCAs, parks and recreation departments, and police athletic leagues. These and many other local agencies offer kids the chance to play together, to develop physical, social, and mental skills, and to develop or maintain fitness while having fun.

Community programs can play an integral part in your child's fitness. As with a good school physical education program, a good community program can have positive lasting effects. Playing a sport in a local league not only can be fun and rewarding, the experience helps your child appreciate being active and fit throughout life.

A quick look at the many benefits community programs have to offer underscores their importance.

Community Programs Do More Than Get Kids Fit

Many families need safe havens for their children after school. Communities are filling this need with expanded after-school programs as well as with supervised sports programs at recreation centers, health clubs, and churches. Stay-at-home parents are also turning to community recreation programs because, in many neighborhoods, rising crime rates have forced parents to rethink the safety of unsupervised pickup games in abandoned lots.

Another new trend is that schools are beginning to coordinate their efforts with community groups. With many school districts cutting back on—or even cutting out—physical education, physical educators are looking to coordinate their resources with outside groups to pick up where they have had to leave off. Local recreation leagues can offset cuts in intramural programs. YMCAs and YWCAs can provide classes for children in diet and nutrition to offset cuts in classroom time spent on this area.

The good news is that these programs are filling gaps; the bad news is that they are not necessarily inclusive. Low-income families and children with working parents may not have the time or money to participate in these programs. The trick is to find out what programs are offered in your community, evaluate them in terms of your child's interests and development, and then sign up!

> **F**itness doesn't just keep you healthy. It also helps keep you off the streets and away from drugs. If you find a sport you enjoy, it can make a real difference in your life.
>
> Bonnie Blair
> *Olympic speed skater*

Community programs bring people together. Once your children get involved, your community will seem smaller and your circle of friends wider.

Community leagues draw people from various social and economic backgrounds. Sport is increasingly available to all children, regardless of sex, race, economic status, or mental or physical ability. Attitudes that may be miles apart in some areas can merge gracefully when children work together as a team.

For example, children may lack knowledge about people with disabilities if they have not had the opportunity to develop the appropriate understanding. Your child will learn to enjoy the camaraderie of disabled children when mainstreaming in youth leagues is done properly. I remember as a child visiting the home of a friend whose brother was mentally retarded. I was amazed at all of the swimming trophies he had. I gained a new respect for him that carried over in non-sports-related areas.

Benchmarks of Good Community Programs

Despite the diversity of their offerings and participants, community programs are united in a few common themes. A good community program revolves around fun. What constitutes fun varies with ages and skill levels. Preschoolers just enjoy the pleasure of movement, while children a little older seek sports for the camaraderie. It's not until later that skill development becomes important. And in some cases, winning is never a factor for sports participation.

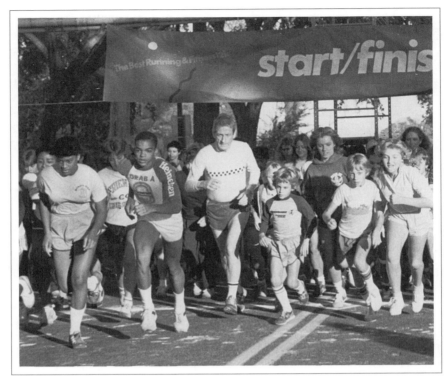

Courtesy of American Running and Fitness Assoc.

Challenge and skill should be balanced to avoid boredom and anxiety. Good programs place kids by developmental age and sports skills, not by chronological age alone. Young children do best in low-key programs that don't require specialized skills, but instead focus on teamwork and movement, such as soccer. Baseball is a good example of a sport meant only for older children: There's a lot of dead time waiting for others at bat, children must master a variety of skills (throwing, batting, and catching) that take time to acquire, and each child's abilities are singled out (when at bat or about to catch the ball), which can increase the stress but not necessarily the fun for a budding young athlete. Children under age 12 should not be expected to practice for their sport more than an hour a day, 3 days a week. Children between 13 and 16 can increase practices to 1-1/2 hours 4 days a week, but no more.

Look for programs that won't pigeonhole your child in a sport or position or require year-round participation. Doing two complementary sports (running and cycling, for example) may help to reduce sports injuries. Likewise, strategies that are useful for one sport, like picks and screens in basketball, are also good for another, like soccer.

The best programs are based on maximum participation. Each child should play at least half of each game. You and your child should be able to voice concerns and opinions to help shape the program to fit your community's needs.

Schools, community recreation departments, and religious organizations can work together to promote a united message so the entire community benefits. Some large cities are developing Inner City Games to enhance community awareness. After the Los Angeles riots in 1992, two of the few areas that were left untouched by the looters were the churches and the recreation centers. These areas transcended the anger of the mobs and symbolized hope for the future. The best programs emphasize good citizenship and academic achievement along with achievement in sport.

> **Parents must make exercising fun for their children. I strongly recommend that parents expose their children to several activities, and let the children choose which of these activities they want to continue participating in.**
>
> Mary Lou Retton
> *Olympic gymnast*

Winning Isn't Everything

Although many community programs are team-oriented, being on a winning team should not be the focal point. There is nothing wrong with winning. Feeling successful and having a sense of accomplishment are good. Yet for every winner there is a loser. Some say that winning only feels as good as losing feels bad. Children don't put an emphasis on winning. It's not even in the top 10 reasons why they compete. Children only feel like losers when they see adults place a high premium on winning.

Community programs that emphasize competition and winning favor early maturers. It is the nature of the sports system developed by adults. Millions of young children begin in sports leagues. As they get older teams become more selective. To make teams competitive, children are asked to practice more and more. Great athletes play, good athletes sit on the bench, and average children are cut. In essence, we are cutting our children right out of a fit lifestyle. This discourages some youngsters from getting involved in sports and physical activity.

One of the benefits of a sports program is exposing children to the facts of life regarding winning and losing and to the stress of competition. If we make losing only a negative experience for our kids we'll almost guarantee that they drop out of sports. My son is used to excelling in many areas. If a sport or skill doesn't come easily or if he loses one too many times, he quickly gets frustrated and refuses to continue. It's hard to motivate him when he thinks he may lose.

What to do? We always encourage our children to do their best. No matter how they perform, but especially when they lose, we need to focus on the positive things that they and the team did during the game. Ask not "Did you win?" but "How'd you play?" Look for well-executed plays or good catches. Build up these aspects of the game, and place the final score as a minor matter. If lots of errors were made, move into this subject gradually. Even if you feel nothing was done right, use the game as a measuring and learning tool by which to measure future performances.

Programs (or parents) that put too much emphasis on winning can put too much stress on young children. Some children are very vulnerable to the negative effects of highly competitive leagues, especially those who already perceive they are not meeting their parents' or coach's expectations. Highly competitive leagues also aren't good for children who base their self-worth on their physical abilities or place too much importance on winning. A child who worries too much about losing probably needs to switch leagues. Help your child work through those fears before placing him in a stressful situation. Few children benefit from a sports program that makes winning the primary goal.

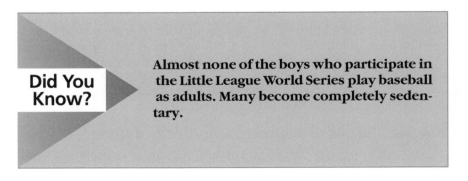

Did You Know?

Almost none of the boys who participate in the Little League World Series play baseball as adults. Many become completely sedentary.

Good Programs Are Around the Corner

Communities have a variety of programs to try out. Each group serves people of various needs and incomes.

Recreation Departments

Because recreation departments are government operated, you and your neighbors can influence the variety and quantity of offerings they provide. Recreation departments offer activities for children from birth on up, educational classes as well as sports instruction. Recreation departments try to address the needs of their community, so many offer after-school programs and provide assistance to children with special needs. There are usually fees charged, but in many communities low-income families can have fees waived or reduced.

To find out what programs are offered in your community, look in the government listing of your phone book under Department of Parks and Recreation. Your library or community center may have information too.

Youth Leagues

Youth leagues are usually developed by local volunteers who determine what sports to offer and for which age groups. If your community doesn't offer the type of program you would like, many national groups will help you start something up locally. You will find a list of such groups at the end of this chapter (see Table 7.5). Some leagues help developing athletes, while others are for more seasoned or competitive types. Be sure you understand the goals of the group before signing your child up.

There is usually a fee involved with joining a league, as well as expenses for equipment or travel. Typical fees run from $15 to $75 a season. Some national groups will offer scholarships to children from low-income families or those with special needs.

If you know the name of your local league, you can look it up in the phone book. However, many leagues are run by volunteers and may not be listed. Your parks and recreation department keeps track of many local leagues, either because their staff supervise the programs or the programs use their fields and gyms. Your child's physical education teacher may be able to recommend a league. Many groups publicize themselves when it's time to register for new seasons. Sporting goods stores often service teams, so they may have a list of contacts as well.

YMCAs, YWCAs, and Other Nonprofit Groups

The types of programs offered by nonprofit organizations vary greatly, depending on the interest and needs of their communities. Many Ys, boys and girls clubs, and religious groups offer programs specifically to help with after-school child care, and they may include fitness in a variety of activities. The good news is that these programs are usually inexpensive and convenient. The bad news is that fitness is not necessarily a priority, and many of the instructors are not trained in fitness activities. If your goal

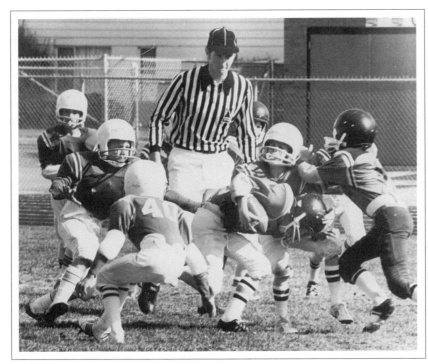

© Doug Brown

is to find a place for your child to enjoy activity, these after-school child care programs are good choices. If your child needs instruction, many Ys also offer exercise classes (such as swimming or martial arts) that are taught by trained professionals. These classes, however, are usually no longer than an hour, so they can't replace after-school care. Fees vary greatly depending on the organization and the type of supervision involved. Low-income families can often get assistance.

Again, the phone book is a good place to start looking for contacts. Try asking friends and neighbors for recommendations. Many community health programs are listed with the local public health department, and the parks and recreation department may again be useful.

Sports Clubs and Schools

Many baby boomers bring their children to the fitness club with them. Some programs, such as KidSports and Gymboree, solely serve children. Other groups that offer instruction for adults in martial arts, tennis, or aerobics have programs for children as well (or allow children to take classes with adults).

Parents who regularly attend fitness clubs will find these programs very convenient. They rarely can serve as child care, because they usually don't last more than an hour. And because they are run by profit-making concerns, fees are always involved and at times can be high. But you often get what you pay for. Instructors are usually certified exercise specialists, with additional training in youth development and motivation.

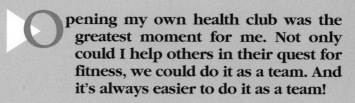

Opening my own health club was the greatest moment for me. Not only could I help others in their quest for fitness, we could do it as a team. And it's always easier to do it as a team!

Richard Simmons
fitness instructor

Look in the yellow pages of your phone book under fitness or health clubs. Ask friends or your child's doctor for suggestions. And check for advertisements in your local paper. Many sporting good stores can assist you in locating quality programs as well.

Now that you have an idea of what community sports programs can offer, let's see how your local programs are faring. Take this quiz and see.

Do You Live in a Fit City?

Here's an easy test to see if your community measures up regarding fitness and if you're using it to its best potential. Answer each question and record how many times each you circle a, b, and c.

1. Does your local recreation department have fitness facilities that children can take advantage of?

    a. yes   b. no   c. I don't know

2. Do you regularly see announcements in your local paper and posted on community billboards alerting you to registration times for youth leagues?

    a. yes   b. no   c. I don't notice

3. Does your church offer sports programs for children?

    a. yes   b. no   c. I don't know

4. Do local schools open up their fitness facilities for community use after school?

    a. yes   b. no   c. I don't know

5. Does the after-school child care program offered by your community include active play time in supervised sports programs?

    a. yes   b. no   c. I don't know

6. Are the coaches in your local youth league required to take classes on coaching techniques for young children?

    a. yes   b. no   c. I don't know

7. Does your community regularly review its parks and recreation department and update and improve facilities as users and needs change?

    a. yes   b. no   c. I don't know

8. Does your school coordinate its efforts with community fitness organizations to be sure that all children get a chance to enjoy a fit lifestyle?

    a. yes   b. no   c. I don't know

9. Do you see access for people with disabilities at your local fitness club?

    a. yes   b. no   c. I haven't thought about it

10. Does your community offer financial aid to low-income families for recreational classes and facilities?

    a. yes   b. no   c. I don't know

✓Scoring

Total the number of a's, b's, and c's.

✓Results

More than six a's—You live in a fit city. Work with your community to be sure your child can take advantage of all it has to offer.

More than five b's—Your city isn't making your job any easier. Contact your local parks and recreation department, city council, and mayor's office as well as your child's physical educator to see if you can assist them in offering better programs. Write a letter to the editor of your local paper highlighting the importance of recreational programs in cities. (Get ammunition from this chapter.)

More than four c's—You aren't taking advantage of one of your best allies. Take some initiative and get informed.

Saturday in the Park— Coaches Make Sports Fun

Of course, you've heard the down side of community programs: coaches and parents pressuring children to perform; fights breaking out at games; lesser skilled children sitting on benches, playing only the minimum time required by the league. Even if these experiences don't turn your child away from being active and fit later in life, they certainly don't promote what community programs are ideally about. A good coach will help your child get an enriching experience from sports and develop a lifelong interest in an active lifestyle.

I helped my mom coach soccer when I was in high school. She was every parent's ideal coach. While she had the skills and knowledge to coach select teams, her favorite team was one with kids from a variety of backgrounds and talents. Each child on her team was unique, and she motivated different kids in different ways. Jennifer was the star, but she had low self-esteem. My mother worked hard to be sure Jennifer didn't feel pressure to carry the team. Darlene, on the other hand, was shy and a beginner. My mom helped Darlene set realistic goals and made sure she participated in practice and in games. To accommodate children with a variety of skills, practices included a smorgasbord of activities so that everyone was challenged and had fun. The girls never chose sides for scrimmages; each team was balanced, and each player tried out a variety of positions.

The father of a player named Marilyn was fiercely competitive. Mom wouldn't tolerate his yelling or derogatory comments and told him if he didn't shape up, he'd have to ship out. At a team meeting with parents, she was applauded for quieting him down. Apparently he'd been the league terror for a number of years, but no one had done anything to neutralize him. Mom was fair, patient, and consistent. She listened to her players and their parents and developed a program where everyone was a winner.

Did You Know?

Ninety percent of the coaches in the U.S. have never taken classes designed to enhance their knowledge of the sports they coach. Many never learn the principles for coaching either.

Safe and Sound Activities

The National Youth Sports Foundation for the Prevention of Athletic Injuries was developed to address the growing number of sports injuries being sustained by children. Each year millions of American children visit family physicians and millions more get treatment in hospital emergency rooms for sports injuries (see Figure 7.1).

Be sure your community program is safe. Requiring a preparticipation physical exam is a sign that the league cares about your child's safety. A good coach can go one step further by giving you a conditioning program for your child at registration time. Being conditioned when the season starts reduces the chance of getting hurt. Ask if your child's coach has taken first aid classes or CPR. If not, perhaps the parents can collect or raise money to help pay for this training (generally about $50). When I coached, I appreciated any help I could get from my parents to enhance my skills.

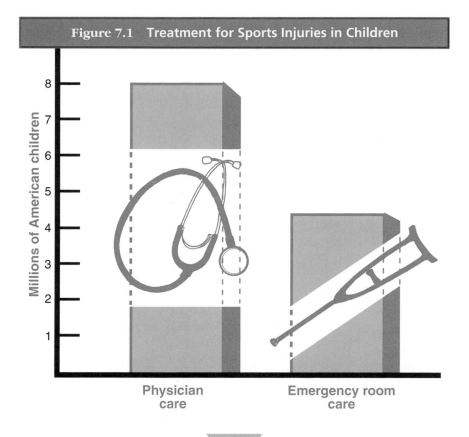

Figure 7.1 Treatment for Sports Injuries in Children

Millions of American children

Physician care

Emergency room care

Coaches who are certified by a national governing body for their sport or one of the national coaching certification programs have the training to reduce injury risks both at practice and at games. A knowledgeable and concerned coach has the team warm up, stretch, and cool down. She also brings a first aid box and ice to practices and games.

Leagues set rules for playing in inclement weather. Games should be postponed during lightning storms, darkness, excessive heat, or excessive cold or if the fields are uneven and unsafe. In any case, if you don't feel the weather or the field is conducive to safe activity, notify the coach that you don't plan to let your child play. Coaches should not encourage children to play in unsafe environments, nor should they chastise any child who does not play.

For more information on guidelines and programs that help make sports safer in your community, contact the National Youth Sports Foundation for the Prevention of Athletic Injuries at 10 Meredith Circle, Needham, MA 02192; phone 617-449-2499.

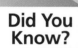

Did You Know?

Gymnastics, ice hockey, and football report the most sports injuries among high school players, according to the National Youth Sports Foundation. Of every 100 girls participating in organized sports, 20 to 22 will get injured. Thirty of every 100 boys get hurt each sports season.

A Team Approach for Coaches and Parents

No matter how great your child's coach is, parental involvement is key. Be sure your child is ready to play. Before the season, schedule your child for a preparticipation physical exam. Tell the doctor what type of play your child will be doing and ask if he is at the right stage in development to enjoy that environment.

Several weeks before the season begins, contact the coach and ask what will be expected physically of your child. Tell the coach about any medical conditions your child has. Ask what risks the coach sees in your child playing and whether there are any conditioning exercises your child can do to help get ready to play.

> **P**lay and physical activity are inextricably linked—not as a task, but as a reward; not as a question, but as an answer; not as a prescription, but as a lifestyle.
>
> George Sheehan, MD
> *runner and author*

Find out what safety equipment is required and make sure your child's equipment is nationally approved. Find out if water will be available at practice and games; if not, provide a jug for your child to take along.

A good coach has at least one parent meeting each season. You may need to reinforce the coach's instructions to your child, so become familiar with the techniques and rules of the game. Help your child find time to practice and make team practices and games. Be sure to notify the coach if your child will miss practice or a game.

Cheering Them On

Your child needs your support. Show that you care about your child's interest in sports by attending as many games, practices, and social events as you can. If you can't be there, ask questions. Remember when important matches are coming up. If you can't attend, see if another family member or a friend can. I always played my best when I knew that someone I cared about (and who cared about me) was watching.

If the youth sports experience is to be a positive one for each child, parents and coaches must demonstrate sportsmanlike behavior. Adults should encourage fun and give lots of praise for little successes along the way. When a child makes a mistake, separate the mistake from the child. (For example, it's not that your child is a bad passer, it's that he threw a bad pass.)

From my coaching days I remember parents who I wanted to keep for every season. They cheered our team whether we won or lost. They knew many of the children's names and called out individual encouragement when it was needed. They participated in team huddles and team cheers. When games were over, they not only praised our team, they also congratulated our opponents. They were great! I will be trying to emulate these star parents when I'm in their shoes.

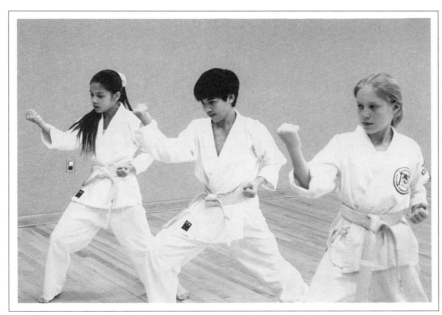

© Doug Brown

Your child's coach and league should not tolerate vulgar language; drugs, alcohol, or cigarettes; berating players; or displaying other negative behavior. With this in mind, be respectful of both coaches and officials at games. Your child will learn good sportsmanship from you. Remain in the spectator area during games, and don't interfere with the coaching. You must be willing to relinquish your parental responsibility to the coach during practices and games (unless, of course, safety is involved). Differences of opinion should be handled calmly and in private.

Between programs at your child's school and within your community, you should be able to find fun activities to keep your child interested and fit. One last area where parents can look for fitness support is the medical community. Look to your child's health care professionals for more than treating chicken pox and colds. They are key in helping you find sports that will complement your child's physical development, and they can help if your child has special needs or becomes injured. The next chapter presents tips on getting the most out of the medical community.

Table 7.5 Sports Organizations

Sport	Organization name and phone	Address	Ages	Sex	Competition	Instruction	Chapters
Archery	National Association of Police Athletic Leagues (407-844-1823)	200 Castlewood Dr., #400 North Palm Beach, FL 33408	6–18	B, G	Yes	Yes	Yes
Badminton	US Badminton Association (719-578-4808)	One Olympic Plaza, Bldg. 10, Rm. 126 Colorado Springs, CO 80809	Open	B, G	Yes	Yes	Yes
Baseball	All American Amateur Baseball Association (614-453-7349)	340 Walker Dr. Zanesville, OH 43701	?–21	B, G	Yes	?	Yes
Baseball	American Amateur Baseball Congress (616-781-2002)	118 Redfield Plaza Marshall, MI 49068	Open	B, G	Yes	?	Yes
Baseball	National Association of Police Athletic Leagues (407-844-1823)	200 Castlewood Dr., #400 North Palm Beach, FL 33408	6–18	B, G	Yes	Yes	Yes
Baseball	American Legion Baseball (317-630-1213)	PO Box 1055 Indianapolis, IN 46206	?–19	?	Yes	?	Yes
Baseball	Dixie Baseball/Softball (615-821-6811)	215 Watauga Ln., PO Box 222 Lookout Mountain, TN 37350	6–12	B	Yes	Yes	Yes
Baseball	George Khoury Association of Baseball Leagues (314-849-8900)	5400 Meramec Bottom Rd. St. Louis, MO 63128	7–?	B, G	?	?	Yes
Baseball	Little League Baseball Inc. (717-326-1921)	PO Box 3485 Williamsport, PA 17701	6–18	B	Yes	Yes	Yes
Baseball	National Amateur Baseball Federation (301-262-5005)	PO Box 705 Bowie, MD 20718	15–18	B	Yes	No	Yes

Sport	Organization	Address	Age	Gender			
Baseball	Pony Baseball, Inc. (412-225-1060)	PO Box 225 Washington, PA 15301	5–18	B	Yes	Yes	Yes
Baseball	Amateur Athletic Union of US (317-872-2900)	3400 W. 86th St. Indianapolis, IN 46268	Open	B, G	Yes	Yes	Yes
Basketball	Biddy Basketball (504-282-0753)	4711 Bancroft Dr. New Orleans, LA 70122	?–12	B, G	Yes	Yes	Yes
Basketball	Sonny Hill Basketball League Inc. (215-474-2801)	429 S. 50th St. Philadelphia, PA 19143	6–18	B, G	Yes	Yes	Yes
Basketball	Youth Basketball of America Inc. (407-363-9262)	PO Box 3067 Orlando, FL 32802	6–18	B, G	Yes	Yes	Yes
Basketball	National Association of Police Athletic Leagues (407-844-1823)	200 Castlewood Dr., #400 North Palm Beach, FL 33408	6–18	B, G	Yes	Yes	Yes
Basketball	Amateur Athletic Union of US (317-872-2900)	3400 W. 86th St. Indianapolis, IN 46268	Open	B, G	Yes	Yes	Yes
Bicycling	League of American Bicyclists (410-539-3399)	190 W. Ostend St., #120 Baltimore, MD 21230-3755	Open	B, G	No	Yes	Yes
Bowling	Young American Bowling Alliance (414-421-4700)	5301 S. 76th St. Greendale, WI 53129	6–21	B, G	Yes	Yes	Yes
Climbing	American Sport Climbers Association (510-376-1640)	35 Greenfield Dr. Moraga, CA 94556	Open	B, G	No	Yes	?
Equestrian	Harness Horse Youth Foundation (317-848-5132)	14950 Greyhound Ct., #210 Carmel, IN 46032	8–18	B, G	?	Yes	?
Equestrian	US Combined Training Association (703-779-0440)	PO Box 2247 Leesburg, VA 22075	Open	B, G	Yes	Yes	?
Fencing	US Fencing Association (719-578-4511)	One Olympic Plaza Colorado Springs, CO 80909	Open	B, G	Yes	Yes	?
Field hockey	US Field Hockey Association (719-578-4587)	One Olympic Plaza Colorado Springs, CO 80909	Open	G	Yes	Yes	?

(continued)

Table 7.5 *(continued)*

Sport	Organization name and phone	Address	Ages	Sex	Competition	Instruction	Chapters
Field hockey	Amateur Athletic Union of US (317-872-2900)	3400 W. 86th St. Indianapolis, IN 46268	Open	B, G	Yes	Yes	Yes
Football	Pop Warner Football (215-752-2691)	586 Middletown Blvd., Ste. C-100 Langhorne, PA 19047	7–15	B	Yes	Yes	Yes
Football	National Association of Police Athletic Leagues (407-844-1823)	200 Castlewood Dr., #400 North Palm Beach, FL 33408	6–18	B, G	Yes	Yes	Yes
Football	US Flag and Touch Football League (216-974-8735)	7709 Ohio St. Mentor, OH 44060	Open	B, G	Yes	Yes	Yes
Golf	American Junior Golf Association (404-998-4653)	2415 Steeplechase Ln. Roswell, GA 30076	11–18	B, G	Yes	Yes	No
Golf	Hook a Kid on Golf (407-684-1141)	2050 Vista Pkway. West Palm Beach, FL 33411	8–14	B, G	Yes	Yes	Yes
Gymnastics	American Trampoline and Tumbling Association (806-637-8670)	1610 E. Cardwell Brownfield, TX 79216	Open	B, G	?	?	?
Gymnastics	USA Gymnastics Federation (317-237-5050)	201 S. Capitol Ave., #300 Indianapolis, IN 46225	Open	B, G	Yes	Yes	Yes
Gymnastics	Amateur Athletic Union of US (317-872-2900)	3400 W. 86th St. Indianapolis, IN 46268	Open	B, G	Yes	Yes	Yes
Handball	US Handball Association (602-795-0434)	2333 N. Tucson Blvd. Tucson, AZ 85716	Open	B, G	Yes	Yes	?

Sport	Organization	Address	Age	Gender			
Handball	US Team Handball Federation (719-578-4582)	One Olympic Plaza Colorado Springs, CO 80909	Open	B, G	Yes	Yes	Yes
Ice hockey	USA Hockey (719-599-5500)	4965 N. 30th St. Colorado Springs, CO 80919	Open	B, G	Yes	Yes	?
Ice skating	Amateur Speedskating Union of the US (708-790-3230)	1033 Shady Ln. Glen Ellyn, IL 60137	Open	B, G	Yes	Yes	?
Ice skating	US Figure Skating Association (719-635-5200)	20 First St. Colorado Springs, CO 80906	Open	B, G	Yes	Yes	?
In-line skating	International In-Line Skating Association (404-728-9707)	PO Box 15482 Atlanta, GA 30333	Open	B, G	Yes	Yes	Yes
Lacrosse	Lacrosse Foundation (410-235-6882)	113 W. University Pkway. Baltimore, MD 21210	Open	B, G	Yes	Yes	Yes
Lacrosse	Lacrosse USA Inc. (303-927-9338)	PO Box 1116 Basalt, CO 81621	Open	B, G	Yes	Yes	Yes
Martial arts	American Amateur Karate Federation (213-483-8261)	1930 Wilshire Blvd., #1208 Los Angeles, CA 90057	Open	B, G	Yes	Yes	Yes
Martial arts	US Taekwondo Union (719-578-4632)	One Olympic Plaza Colorado Springs, CO 80909	Open	B, G	Yes	Yes	Yes
Martial arts	National Association of Police Athletic Leagues (407-844-1823)	200 Castlewood Dr., #400 North Palm Beach, FL 33408	6–18	B, G	Yes	Yes	Yes
Martial arts	Amateur Athletic Union of US (317-872-2900)	3400 W. 86th St. Indianapolis, IN 46268	Open	B, G	Yes	Yes	Yes
Orienteering	US Orienteering Federation (404-363-2110)	PO Box 1444 Forest Park, GA 30051	Open	B, G	Yes	Yes	Yes
Paddle tennis	US Paddle Tennis Association (213-856-6367)	Box 30 Culver City, CA 90232	Open	B, G	Yes	Yes	Yes
Racquetball	American Amateur Racquetball Association (719-635-5396)	1685 W. Uintah Colorado Springs, CO 80904	Open	B, G	Yes	Yes	Yes

(continued)

Table 7.5 (continued)

Sport	Organization name and phone	Address	Ages	Sex	Competition	Instruction	Chapters
Rodeo	National High School Rodeo Association (303-452-0820)	11178 N. Huron, #7 Denver, CO 80234	14–18	B, G	Yes	Yes	Yes
Rodeo	National Little Britches Rodeo Association (719-389-0333)	1045 W. Rio Grande Colorado Springs, CO 80906	8–18	B, G	Yes	Yes	Yes
Roller skating	Roller Skating Confederation (402-483-7551)	PO Box 6579 Lincoln, NE 68506	Open	B, G	Yes	Yes	Yes
Rowing	US Rowing Association (317-237-5656)	201 S. Capitol Ave., #400 Indianapolis, IN 46225	Open	B, G	Yes	Yes	Yes
Rugby	US Rugby Football Foundation (617-426-7799)	1 Beacon St., 24th Fl. Boston, MA 02108	Open	B, G	Yes	Yes	?
Rugby	US Rugby Union (719-637-1022)	3595 E. Fountain Blvd. Colorado Springs, CO 80910	Open	B, G	Yes	Yes	Yes
Running	American Running & Fitness Association (301) 913-9517	4405 East West Highway #405 Bethesda, MD 20814	Open	B, G	No	Yes	No
Running	Road Runner's Club of America (703-836-0558)	1150 S. Washington St., Ste. 250 Alexandria, VA 22314	Open	B, G	Yes	Yes	Yes
Running	Amateur Athletic Union of US (317-872-2900)	3400 W. 86th St. Indianapolis, IN 46268	Open	B, G	Yes	Yes	Yes
Skiing	US Recreational Ski Association (714-634-1050)	1315 E. Pacifico Ave. Anaheim, CA 92805	Open	B, G	Yes	Yes	Yes

Sport	Organization	Age	Gender			
Skiing	US Ski Association 1500 Kearns Blvd., PO Box 100 Park City, UT 84060 (801-649-9090)	Open	B, G	Yes	Yes	Yes
Soccer	American Youth Soccer Organization 5403 W. 138th St. Hawthorne, CA 90250 (310-643-6455)	6–18	B, G	Yes	Yes	Yes
Soccer	Soccer Association for Youth 4903 Vine St. Cincinnati, OH 45217 (513-242-4263)	6–18	B, G	Yes	Yes	Yes
Soccer	US Soccer Federation 1801-11 S. Prairie Ave. Chicago, IL 60616 (312-808-1300)	Open	B, G	Yes	Yes	Yes
Soccer	National Association of Police Athletic Leagues 200 Castlewood Dr., #400 North Palm Beach, FL 33408 (407-844-1823)	6–18	B, G	Yes	Yes	Yes
Soccer	US Youth Soccer Association 2050 N. Plano, #100 Richardson, TX 75082 (214-235-4499)	6–18	B, G	Yes	Yes	Yes
Soccer	Soccer in the Streets 211 Porter Ln. Jonesboro, GA 30236 (404-477-0354)	6–19	B, G	Yes	Yes	Yes
Soccer	Amateur Athletic Union of US 3400 W. 86th St. Indianapolis, IN 46268 (317-872-2900)	Open	B, G	Yes	Yes	Yes
Softball	Dixie Baseball/Softball 215 Watauga Ln., PO Box 222 Lookout Mountain, TN 37350 (615-821-6811)	6–18	G	Yes	Yes	Yes
Softball	Little League Baseball Inc. PO Box 3485 Williamsport, PA 17701 (717-326-1921)	6–18	G	Yes	Yes	Yes
Softball	National Association of Police Athletic Leagues 200 Castlewood Dr., #400 North Palm Beach, FL 33408 (407-844-1823)	6–18	B, G	Yes	Yes	Yes
Softball	Pony Baseball, Inc. PO Box 225 Washington, PA 15301 (412-225-1060)	5–18	G	Yes	Yes	Yes
Softball	Amateur Softball Association of America 2801 NE 50th St. Oklahoma City, OK 73111 (405-424-5266)	Open	B, G	Yes	Yes	Yes
Softball	Cinderella Softball League Inc. PO Box 1411 Corning, NY 14830 (607-937-5469)	6–18	G	Yes	Yes	Yes

(continued)

Table 7.5 (continued)

Sport	Organization name and phone	Address	Ages	Sex	Competition	Instruction	Chapters
Softball	Amateur Athletic Union of US (317-872-2900)	3400 W. 86th St. Indianapolis, IN 46268	Open	B, G	Yes	Yes	Yes
Squash	National Squash Tennis Association (212-661-2070)	50 Vanderbilt Ave. New York, NY 10017	?	B, G	Yes	Yes	Yes
Surfing	National Scholastic Surfing Association (310-592-2140)	PO Box 495 Huntington Beach, CA 92648	6-18	B, G	Yes	Yes	Yes
Swimming	US Swimming, Inc. (719-578-4578)	One Olympic Plaza Colorado Springs, CO 80909	Open	B, G	Yes	Yes	Yes
Swimming	US Synchronized Swimming (317-237-5700)	201 S. Capitol Ave., #510 Indianapolis, IN 46225	Open	B, G	Yes	Yes	Yes
Swimming	National Association of Police Athletic Leagues (407-844-1823)	200 Castlewood Dr., #400 North Palm Beach, FL 33408	6-18	B, G	Yes	Yes	Yes
Swimming	US Diving (317-237-5252)	201 S. Capitol Ave., #430 Indianapolis, IN 46225	Open	B, G	Yes	Yes	Yes
Swimming	Amateur Athletic Union of US (317-872-2900)	3400 W. 86th St. Indianapolis, IN 46268	Open	B, G	Yes	Yes	Yes
Table tennis	US Table Tennis (800-326-8788)	One Olympic Plaza Colorado Springs, CO 80909	Open	B, G	Yes	Yes	Yes
Table tennis	Amateur Athletic Union of US (317-872-2900)	3400 W. 86th St. Indianapolis, IN 46268	Open	B, G	Yes	Yes	Yes

Sport	Organization	Address	Age	Gender			
Tennis	US Tennis Association (914-696-7000)	70 W. Red Oak Ln. White Plains, NY 10604	Open	B, G	Yes	Yes	Yes
Tennis	National Association of Police Athletic Leagues (407-844-1823)	200 Castlewood Dr., #400 North Palm Beach, FL 33408	6–18	B, G	Yes	Yes	Yes
Track and field	USA Track & Field (317-261-0500)	One Hoosier Dome, #140 Indianapolis, IN 46225	10–18	B, G	Yes	Yes	Yes
Track and field	Amateur Athletic Union of US (317-872-2900)	3400 W. 86th St. Indianapolis, IN 46268	Open	B, G	Yes	Yes	Yes
Volleyball	USA Volleyball Association (719-637-8300)	3595 E. Fountain Blvd., #I-2 Colorado Springs, CO 80910	Open	B, G	Yes	Yes	Yes
Volleyball	Amateur Athletic Union of US (317-872-2900)	3400 W. 86th St. Indianapolis, IN 46268	Open	B, G	Yes	Yes	Yes
Water skiing	American Water Ski Association (813-324-4341)	799 Overlook Dr. Winter Haven, FL 33884	Open	B, G	Yes	Yes	Yes
Weight lifting	Amateur Athletic Union of US (317-872-2900)	3400 W. 86th St. Indianapolis, IN 46268	Open	B, G	Yes	Yes	Yes
Wrestling	USA Wrestling (719-598-8181)	6155 Lehman Dr. Colorado Springs, CO 80918	Open	B	Yes	Yes	Yes
Wrestling	Amateur Athletic Union of US (317-872-2900)	3400 W. 86th St. Indianapolis, IN 46268	Open	B, G	Yes	Yes	Yes

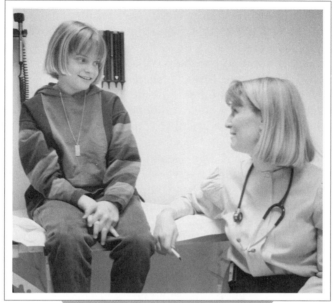

© Doug Brown

8

The Medical Team for Fitness

Most people associate the medical community with the treatment of illnesses and injuries. But the growing trend is to focus not only on treatment but also on prevention. Health care professionals can help steer your child toward activities that will complement her physical development and health.

The medical community can help enhance your child's sports experiences and healthy lifestyle. Physicians aren't the only professionals who can help with your child's fitness and health: Dietitians, psychologists, physical therapists, and athletic trainers are being sought more and more—often teaming up with physicians—to guide children's sports participation.

Still, you need to be in charge. Health care professionals are in practice to serve you and your child's needs, not to dictate what those needs are. The key lies in figuring out just how they can help you meet those needs. Let's look at the role the medical community plays in children's fitness.

How Your Doctor Can Help

Your doctor's job is to keep your child healthy. The doctor should begin counseling on diet and activity recommendations at your child's first visit—and continue throughout your child's life.

Aside from general health recommendations, your doctor should detect conditions that may limit your child's ability to be physically active or predispose him to sports injury. Thoughtful exams can root out potential problems. It is never a reasonable solution to stop all physical activity for a long period. Even cancer patients improve their strength and mental health through supervised exercise. Always look for alternatives if your child runs into a barrier in athletic pursuits. If your son develops "Little League elbow" (tendinitis), for example, he can take up soccer. If your daughter has asthma, swimming is a wonderful sport to pursue. Even children who use wheelchairs can benefit from exercise. There's even wheelchair basketball and tennis! Get a second opinion if your doctor says your child must stop a sport that means a lot to her.

You can also get advice from your doctor on health-related issues such as diet, stress reduction, and substance abuse.

As your child matures your doctor should talk with the two of you about weight control and nutrition; avoiding sports injuries; tobacco, alcohol, and drug use; wearing seat belts; breast and testicle self-examination; and birth control.

Your doctor also should keep you apprised of your child's maturity level. A pediatrician sees many children daily and is a good source of objective

Did You Know?

Fewer than 30% of doctors say they counsel their patients regarding fitness or nutrition.

information on where your child stands in relation to peers. Both physical and mental maturity need to be considered. Prepare your child for this type of evaluation. Many find it embarrassing, so it helps to be forewarned.

Children who are regularly asked to perform above their maturity level get injured more easily. Their self-esteem also suffers when they can't perform at that unrealistic level. Talk with your pediatrician about sports options that your child will enjoy and benefit from.

Choosing a Doctor for Your Child

A good family doctor can make an enormous impact on your child's health, yet most people spend little time or effort choosing a physician. The changes in our health care system mean that many consumers are allowed fewer choices of doctors. This makes it doubly important that you review your options carefully.

Sports medicine, fitness, and preventive medicine are not specialties that can be studied in medical school. There is, however, a new certificate of qualification available to pediatricians, family practice physicians, emergency physicians, and geriatric physicians. This certificate means the doctor is familiar with health promotion strategies as well as injury prevention and treatment. You will be able to find more doctors with this certificate in the coming years. Pediatricians and family physicians can also be members of sports medicine subgroups within their medical societies.

How can you tell if your doctor will be a key player on your family fitness team? Ask if the physician counsels patients on diet and exercise. Few do—seek out ones that will. Is your doctor physically active? Medical students are taught little about exercise and nutrition. Physicians who are knowledgeable often have learned because of a personal interest.

Look around your doctor's office for signs of involvement in sports medicine organizations. You may see certificates from medical societies your doctor belongs to. Are there any sports medicine publications in the waiting room?

If the only doctors you can find solely treat disease and can't foster your child's fitness, look for allied professionals who can help. Physician assistants and nurse practitioners often have more time to talk with patients than a physician does and are typically more knowledgeable about improving children's health through diet and exercise. Progressive doctors recognize their weaknesses and develop close ties with nutritionists, psychologists, athletic trainers, and therapists.

While your doctor may not be able to counsel you personally on specifics, she or he should refer you to these other professionals who can. Seek out a physician like this.

Did You Know?

According to Michael Goran, PhD, most doctors recommend diets that contain more calories than children really need. The World Health Organization recommends a diet of 1,800 calories a day, when in fact, Goran has found that most children only burn about 1,400 calories a day.

Pediatrician or Family Practitioner?

Both pediatricians and family practitioners are specialists trained to treat children. However, pediatricians are immersed in children; 100% of their time is devoted to kids and their ailments. So in many cases, pediatricians are recommended up through puberty.

The down side of using pediatricians is that few know anything about sports medicine or health promotion. More family practitioners are beginning to counsel both parents and children in this area. Family practitioners also know the entire family, which can help when emotional or stressful situations arise. Family physicians may have either DO (doctor of osteopathy) or MD (doctor of medicine) as a degree.

Other Health Consultants

Whom should you see if your child develops a sport injury? Check first with your child's doctor. But if the injury is slow in healing or your doctor recommends it, see a sports medicine professional. Which one? It depends on the injury (see Table 8.1).

Table 8.1	Medical Specialists Who Treat Sports Injuries
Injury site	Specialist (degree in parentheses)
Arms/legs	Orthopedists (MD), physiatrists—physical medicine and rehabilitation doctors (MD), osteopaths (DO)
Back	Orthopedists (MD), osteopaths (DO), chiropractors (DC)
Feet	Podiatrists (DPM), orthopedists (MD), physiatrists (MD), osteopaths (DO)
Joints	Orthopedists (MD), physiatrists (MD), osteopaths (DO)

In some states, sports injuries can be initially diagnosed and treated by allied professionals, such as sport physical therapists (they have RPT after their names) and athletic trainers (who have ATC after their names). Physical therapists who belong to the sports medicine section of the American Physical Therapy Association and all athletic trainers are specialists in helping treat and prevent sports injuries, and they often work with high schools and recreation departments.

You may also want to consult with professionals in other areas. A nutritionist can help you develop and monitor your child's diet. The suffix RD means that a nutritionist is a registered dietitian with the American Dietetic Association. This professional society also has a sports and cardiovascular nutrition section to help athletes of any age. Children with eating disorders or kids having a hard time coping with stress can benefit from psychological help. You don't necessarily need to see a psychiatrist (MD), however. Ask your family doctor for a referral to a psychologist (MS or PhD) or a clinical social worker (LCSW or MSW).

Questions for Your Child's Next Checkup

An effective relationship with your doctor requires two-way communication. My friend Jane, who is a pediatrician and mom, told me about a young patient with a sensitivity to salt. Even though the boy's family had stopped using salt at home, the child wasn't getting better, and Jane was getting frustrated. Finally his mother mentioned that her son was going through close to a bottle a week of soy sauce (which is very high in sodium). Doctors can't help us unless they know all of the facts.

njuries were one of the toughest things for me to overcome while I was competing in gymnastics. The healing process was so frustrating because I was always anxious to get back to my workouts right away.

Mary Lou Retton
Olympic gymnast

Here are some questions you should ask your doctor so that together you can help your child be successful, fit, and happy.

1. *What is my child's developmental age?* Successful sports programs are geared toward your child's developmental, not chronological, age.

2. *How does she compare to her peers?* Help your child cope with any weaknesses. Your child wants to feel successful and competent among peers.

3. *What common problems occur in children this age?* Every age is blessed with certain talents and hurdles. Most pediatricians have seen it all and have come to know what works and what doesn't.

4. *Can you recommend activities that will help my child improve any weaknesses he may have?* Your child is always changing and can always improve in some way. No child should be indelibly labeled clumsy or slow. The trick is finding out what is needed and finding a fun way to help your child improve.

5. *Should I restrict any activities? Why?* Physical or mental limitations may make it necessary for you to curtail specific activities. Sometimes overzealous or well-meaning parents have a hard time determining what a child can handle. Your doctor should be able to give objective advice based on work with many children. If your doctor says your child must stop an activity, however, ask why, and look for an alternative your child will enjoy.

6. *What should my child be eating at this time? How many calories should she be consuming?* Nutritional needs vary with age and activity level. Many parents think their children need to eat more than they really do.

7. When should we reschedule a checkup? What will be done at that time? Regular visits to your child's doctor will keep everyone up-to-date. By checking on what to do next and when, you can be sure to include these important visits into your busy schedule. Almost any schedule can be changed if you plan ahead.

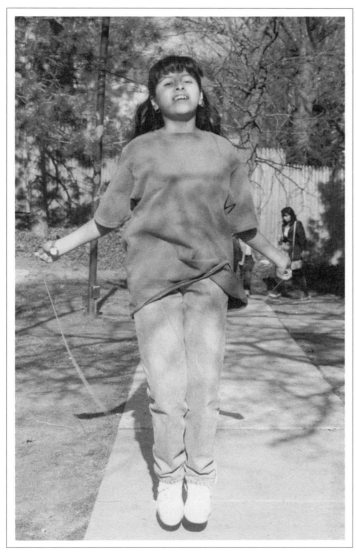

© Doug Brown

Getting Cleared for Sports Participation

Many states require annual physical evaluations before children can play team sports. If your state doesn't, have it done anyway. But don't use a preparticipation screening as your child's only annual checkup. It rarely includes health screening and immunizations your child may need. You can combine the two types of exams if you make it clear you want both when scheduling an appointment.

Your school or recreation department may schedule specific times and places for preparticipation exams. Give your pediatrician a copy of the results. If your community doesn't offer these exams, have your child's doctor do one.

There are pros and cons to both situations. Your pediatrician will be able to rely on close familiarity with your child and your family when reviewing your child's health status. Your child's doctor is also more likely than the people staffing community-run, station-based screening programs to counsel you on ways to improve health. And this approach is more private than community screenings, so an easily embarrassed teen may prefer it.

On the other hand, many family physicians are less aware of sports medicine problems. They may not have the facilities to test performance either. They also don't always know what is expected of them by the school athletic staff. And a physician visit usually costs more than a community-based screening.

Elements of the Preparticipation Exam

A variety of areas are checked in a preparticipation exam, including

- blood pressure,
- diet,
- eyes,
- heart,
- height and weight,
- lungs,
- maturity level,
- medical history,
- preexisting problems,
- pulse, and
- skin.

Your child is checked for any condition that will increase her risk of being injured in sports or that could increase the risk of injury to others. If a condition is discovered, find out whether your child needs specific medication, equipment, or training to participate safely. Also ask if limited participation can be allowed while treatment is being initiated.

Doctors also evaluate whether a given sport is too rough for a particular child. Smaller children shouldn't be allowed to play contact sports with kids who are bigger than they are. Certain medical conditions also preclude a child's playing contact sports, such as having one kidney, carditis, an enlarged liver or spleen, instability in the neck, or poorly controlled convulsions or seizures. Endurance level is also assessed to be sure a child is fit enough to play the sport. A child with an enlarged spleen, for example, can only enjoy moderately strenuous and nonstrenuous activities. Otherwise, developmental maturity will be the guide.

The American Academy of Pediatrics classifies sports to help doctors select appropriate activities for children. Noncontact sports are most suitable for young or small children. The more contact in a sport, the more important it is to have a trained coach or teacher present. Another consideration is the sport's intensity. Beginners (at any age) should look toward less strenuous sports; as their fitness levels progress, the intensity of their sports can too. Children placed in sports that do not suit their physical condition are likely to get hurt or become disenchanted with sports. Tables 8.2 and 8.3 rate sports on their levels of contact and strenuousness.

Table 8.2 What's a Contact Sport?		
Contact or collision	**Limited contact or impact**	**Noncontact**
• Boxing	• Baseball	• Aerobic dance
• Field hockey	• Basketball	• Archery
• Football	• Bicycling	• Badminton
• Ice hockey	• Diving	• Crew/rowing
• Lacrosse	• Gymnastics	• Fencing
• Martial arts	• Handball	• Golf
• Rodeo	• Horseback riding	• Swimming
• Soccer	• Racquetball	• Tennis
• Wrestling	• Skating	• Track
	• Skiing	• Weight lifting
	• Softball	
	• Squash	
	• Track and field	
	• Volleyball	

Reprinted from Pediatrics (1988).

Table 8.3 How Strenuous Is a Sport?		
Strenuous	**Moderately strenuous**	**Not strenuous**
• Aerobic dance • All contact sports* • Crew/rowing • Swimming • Tennis • Track and field • Weight lifting	• Badminton • Curling • Fencing • Table tennis	• Archery • Golf • Riflery

*See Table 8.2 for a listing of common contact sports.

What If Your Child Overdoes It?

Your child may develop a sports injury even if you have been very careful in matching the activity to your child's development. There is a fine line between stressing the body to improve and stressing it so much it gets hurt. Most recreational athletes develop some type of sports injury that affects their training. Youthful exuberance doesn't help the matter. If your child complains of soreness after exercise, suggest that he cut back a bit for a day or two to allow his muscles to repair and strengthen.

Prescribing ARICE

Sporadic soreness comes with an active lifestyle. But if your child complains of soreness after every workout session or even during workouts, it is time for ARICE—antiinflammatants, rest, ice, compression, and elevation are the best way to treat overuse injuries.

Antiinflammatants

When a muscle, bone, or joint gets hurt, the body sends in a work crew to start healing the trauma. In most cases the body sends too much help for the space and the area becomes swollen. Antiinflammatory medications reduce this swelling. Look for medications made with ibuprofen in your local drugstore to not only reduce swelling but also cut the pain of an injury. Children over age 10 who do not have flu symptoms can take aspirin, which also does the trick. In specific cases, your doctor may prescribe a stronger, antiinflammatory medication.

Rest

It's important to stop stressing the muscle, bone, or joint that hurts. If the injury just began, your child can try her luck the next day at half effort. If it hurts a lot or if she has been ignoring it, she needs to stay off the injured area for 3 days to 2 weeks. That doesn't means she needs bed rest; just avoid stressing the painful area. A different sport that doesn't hurt (swimming usually is fine except in the case of shoulder pain) or one that isn't as stressful (walking instead of running, for example) can be continued. The main idea is to do something that doesn't cause pain either during or after activity.

Ice

Ice wrapped in a towel or put inside an ice pack or plastic zipper bag should be placed on the newly injured area to reduce swelling. You can also keep reusable gel packs in the freezer. Don't let the ice sit directly on the skin, and remove it after 15 minutes (sooner if the area feels tingly). Gently massaging the ice around the area works well too. Ice should be applied to an injured area two or three times a day.

Compression

When possible, the injured area should be wrapped with an elastic bandage or a special sleeve that compresses the joint. Some wraps also cool the area at the same time—a double bonus—but they should be removed after 15 minutes. Wrapping, like icing and antiinflammatants, helps reduce swelling.

Elevation

The injured area should be raised if possible to stop blood from pooling.

If your child's injury isn't better after about a week of ARICE, contact a sports medicine professional for further advice. If the injury seems to be on the mend, your child can return to activities. Depending on the degree of injury or how long the injury took to heal, you may want to have your child put warm compresses on the injured area right before working out and cold compresses after practice.

Did You Know?

Acetaminophen (found in Tylenol and other products) is not an antiinflammatant. Acetaminophen cuts pain but not swelling.

Traumatic Injury

Overuse injuries usually creep up over time. Traumatic injuries occur suddenly, perhaps because your child gets hit or falls. You should contact your doctor for many instances of traumatic injury.

Bumps and Bruises

Most bumps and bruises respond well to ice. Some may need an antiinflammatant to reduce swelling and pain.

Cuts

Your first goal with a cut is to stop the bleeding. Most cuts will stop bleeding if you gently compress them. If bleeding doesn't stop within 10 minutes of compression, call your doctor. Once bleeding is stopped, the next step is to clean the wound with an antiseptic. Then cover it with a bandage until night. At night expose the wound to the air to dry. Only cover it again if your child will get it dirty.

Sprains and Strains

If your child falls or gets kicked and finds it difficult or painful to move a joint, it is probably strained or sprained. In most cases, compressing the injured area with an elastic bandage, applying ice for 10 to 20 minutes three or four times a day, and administering antiinflammatants will help. Even so, take your child to the doctor to rule out a broken bone—often a sprain and a broken bone will produce similar symptoms. Your doctor will probably wrap the injury to keep it stable and compress the swelling.

After 1 to 3 weeks, your child will start stretching and strengthening exercises. Warm, moist compresses are also used to stimulate blood flow. Gel packs are portable (so your child can apply the heat anywhere at any time) and easy to recharge (by heating in the microwave or on top of the stove). Depending on the injury, your child can be back on the field in 1 to 6 weeks.

Broken Bones

If your child can't put weight on the injured area or can't bend a joint, a bone may be broken. But long-term nagging pain is also a symptom of a break. An easy fall can result in a broken bone, so don't underestimate the importance of seeing a doctor. X-rays are often needed to determine the existence of a break and how to set it. It may be that casting is only required for a week or two, but bad breaks can take 6 to 8 weeks in a cast, with physical therapy following.

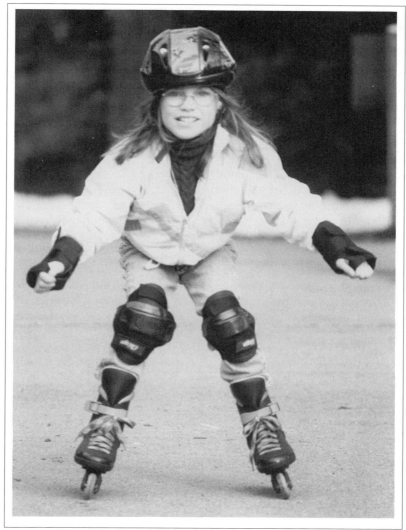

© Doug Brown

Head, Neck, and Back Injuries

Never underestimate the danger of an injury to the head, neck, or back. If your child has trouble moving after an injury, do not encourage movement. Instead, call 911 and stabilize her so she can't move. Do not lift her head onto a pillow. Just try to keep her warm and immobile until help arrives. If your child can move normally, check her eyes by shining a light in them. Do the pupils dilate? If not, take her to a hospital. If she seems okay, call your doctor, explain the incident, and do as the doctor suggests.

Conditions Affecting Exercise and Sports

Almost all of us, whatever our state of health or fitness, benefit from exercise. But some people do need a little more support and planning to get started on a fitness program. Here are a few common conditions that require special attention.

Diabetes

Diabetes is a condition in which the body does not properly balance blood sugar levels. Exercise helps diabetic children. Obesity, often a problem among kids with diabetes, can be reduced with exercise. And combining exercise and good diet helps reduce the amount of insulin a diabetic child needs.

Because exercise increases the rate at which glucose is removed from the blood, a child with diabetes needs to balance insulin and carbohydrate intake with any physical activity. You and your child should work closely with a doctor or nurse-educator to learn how to monitor this interaction. Usually extensive exercise should be avoided during peak insulin activity, which is about 2 to 4 hours after an insulin injection.

Generally speaking, there is no sport that a person with diabetes should have problems pursuing given proper supervision. A number of Olympic and professional athletes have diabetes. Let your doctor know the type and intensity of activity your child is interested in. Diabetes is only a problem when proper precautions are not taken. If activity is new to your child, you may need to monitor the initial activity very closely.

Once you and your doctor have worked out a game plan, contact your child's exercise leader or coach to explain your child's condition. Your doctor may have educational materials you can share with your child's coach or physical educator. Be sure your child's activity is supervised by someone who is prepared to help out in an emergency. For more information contact the International Diabetic Athletes Association, 1647 W. Bethany Home Rd., #B, Phoenix, AZ 85015; phone 602-433-2113.

> **N**othing makes you prouder than coming back and being your best. One of my greatest achievements was my first day back from injury on opening day with the White Sox. I hit a home run! All my hard work and discipline paid off the moment I saw that ball soar through the sky.
>
> Bo Jackson
> *former professional baseball player*
> *(Chicago White Sox)*

Asthma

During an asthma attack, the airways suddenly get smaller, making breathing difficult. The condition can be caused by a variety of factors, from pollution to exercise. Even so, studies show that people with asthma benefit from exercise because it makes their lungs stronger and better able to carry on vigorous daily activities. Asthma can be controlled with medication and should not hamper exercise.

Did You Know?

In the 1984 Olympic Games, 67 athletes had asthma—and 41 of them won medals!

If your child has asthma, talk with your doctor about the sports your child will be pursuing, how often, and at what intensity. With this information your doctor can prescribe the appropriate medication and dosages. Usually taking the proper medication before exercise can reduce or eliminate asthma symptoms. Warming up before starting vigorous activity is always important, but even more so for a child with asthma.

Warm-ups should be longer and more gradual. Because warm, moist air often reduces the chances of an attack, swimming is a common sport of choice for people with asthma. However, all sports are possible with proper control.

Alert your child's physical educator, exercise leader, or coach regarding his condition, and provide information about asthma and your child's needs. Be sure the adult is willing and able to help out in case of an emergency (but also be sure that the person realizes that emergencies are not likely if your child is supervised thoughtfully). Your child may need to take medication before or during exercise. If your child is too young to take on these responsibilities, be sure the exercise leader is willing and able to stand in.

Obesity

Many people do not realize that children who are obese have special needs when it comes to exercise. Although exercise is key to fitness improvement, overweight children often are neglected in physical education class and not encouraged to participate in after-school athletic activities. This is wrong! Children who are obese have a number of problems, and many of them can be helped by activity. Not only will exercise burn additional calories and tone muscles, if supervised correctly it will boost self-esteem—often at a low point for kids who are obese. But if activity is supervised incorrectly, an obese child may be turned off to sports with a vengeance and possibly never try again. Be sure to review the information in chapter 4 on maintaining a healthy weight and on working with your school in chapter 6. A good teacher can be quite an asset in motivating an overweight child.

If your child is obese, consult with your doctor regarding your plans to make physical activity a part of life. Discuss the types of sports your child is interested in and ask if there are any limitations or guidelines your physician can suggest.

In general, an obese child does best in non-weight-bearing exercises. Exercises that stress bones and joints may be too much. Likewise, intensity and duration of workouts should be increased gradually to reduce chances of injury. Sports like hiking, bicycling, swimming, and martial arts are often good choices.

Another concern is heat. Children in general don't handle heat well, and a child who is obese is at greater risk for overheating. Be sure your child is closely supervised when exercising in hot weather. Be extra careful if the temperature tops 65 degrees Fahrenheit.

A common myth is that obese children have poor endurance. Generally adults who are obese have poor endurance because of years of neglect, but heavy children aren't the same. Studies have shown that overweight children often have the same oxygen uptake as their lighter weight counterparts. Vigorous activity is usually safe and effective for them.

Amenorrhea

Another condition that you should be aware of if you have a daughter is amenorrhea, or the absence of menstruation. It is not uncommon for athletically competitive young women to start their periods in their late teens. In most cases, this is not a problem. Researchers are not sure why menstruation is delayed, but some suspect it is due to insufficient nutrition. Keep your family physician aware of your daughter's menstrual status. If she hasn't had a first period by age 17 or 18, tests are warranted. A number of older female athletes are amenorrheic (do not menstruate). This is an unhealthy state that can weaken the bones and may lead to osteoporosis, a bone-thinning disease.

Children With Challenges

The world is not an easy place for children. But some children have an especially tough time. Those with physical or mental limitations are often forced to work doubly hard in a world that often does not understand their true abilities. Parents of children with disabilities may also have a tough time. They want to push their children to achieve, yet they don't want to expect so much that they hurt their children's self-esteem. But there is good news. Many barriers for the disabled are being broken. Physically challenged individuals are really just that—challenged, not handicapped. Many limitations once imposed on children with disabilities are being proven unnecessary or even harmful. Almost every child can benefit from a physical activity and sports program.

Did You Know?

Six of every 10 disabled persons polled had not engaged in a recreational or leisure activity during the previous year because of the disability.

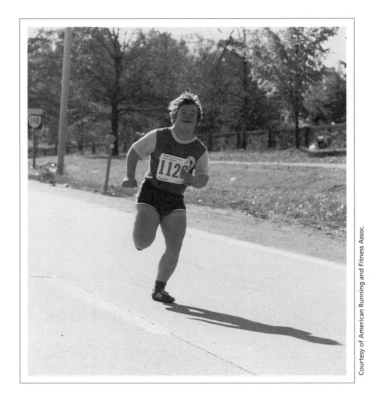

Courtesy of American Running and Fitness Assoc.

Parental Support for the Child With a Disability

If your child has a handicapping condition, she needs your guidance, love, support, and enthusiasm. Special Olympics, an organization that helps thousands of mentally retarded children each year learn the joys of sports, has a special division just to help parents help their children. Their advice is worthwhile for parents of children with any type of disability:

▼ Focus on skill development, not on winning.

▼ Allow sports to help your child learn more about his abilities and test his boundaries. Let him risk failure as well as success.

▼ Be honest with your child's coach or exercise leader. Only by working together will you make a positive impact on your child's development.

▼ Focus on what your child does well. Help her see what she has mastered and let her know you are proud. Many handicapped children want so much to succeed (to please you or their coach) that they lose sight of the fun factor themselves.

▼ Sports should help your child learn to set personal goals (not parental goals) and attain them personally (not through nagging or through threats). If you feel you must be negative with your child, something is wrong. Talk with his coach. Ask him if he's having fun. Is this the right sport? Your child should be participating because he wants to, not out of pressure or guilt.

▼ Help your child work through her fears or anxiety. What might seem like a molehill to you could be a mountain to your child. Talk out her fears, and express your confidence and support.

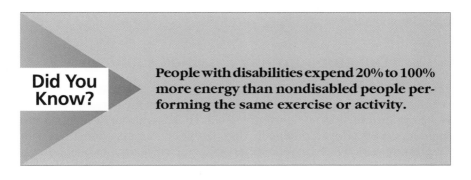

Did You Know?

People with disabilities expend 20% to 100% more energy than nondisabled people performing the same exercise or activity.

Children With Physical Disabilities

Many children with physical disabilities are discouraged from participating in fitness activities not so much because of the disability but because of a low level of fitness. By participating in carefully designed fitness programs, however, these children can get stronger, build their endurance, and enjoy more active lifestyles. Increased fitness helps children with physical disabilities participate in more mainstream activities and become less dependent on others.

It is nearly impossible to say what sports are inaccessible to physically disabled children. Wheelchair users have been known to go rappelling! Talk with your doctor about the options available to your disabled child. The end of this chapter lists national organizations that can provide you with information and referrals to local leagues and coaches.

Although athletes with disabilities may not be injured any more often than their nondisabled peers, the types of injuries they sustain are usually specific to their disabilities and sports. Wheelchair athletes, for example, are more likely than others to develop problems from exercising in extremely hot or cold temperatures. Also common are overuse injuries from inadequate training or warm-up, blisters, cuts and bruises from falls or contact sports, pressure sores, carpal tunnel syndrome, and muscle soreness.

Breaking Barriers

The Americans with Disabilities Act of 1990 is the nation's first comprehensive civil rights law for people with disabilities. It aims to eliminate discrimination against people with physical or mental disabilities. In general, no organization can deny disabled individuals the right to participate, treat them unequally, or separate them from nondisabled individuals. Organizations are asked to make reasonable modifications to their policies, practices, and procedures in order to make their programs available to people with disabilities. Only if the modification would fundamentally alter the nature of the goods or services can this requirement be waived.

Developmentally Disabled Children

There are mutual benefits when retarded children participate in noncompetitive sports with children of average intelligence. One important benefit is the opportunity for the nondisabled child to learn about disabilities and their effects on a developmentally disabled peer. Parents of children with mental retardation need to remember one of the cornerstones of children's fitness: Developmental age is more important than chronological age. Keep in mind persistence, attention span, emotional control, and ability to understand the rules of the game when mainstreaming your child.

Children with mental retardation often prefer games over simple exercises. Even so, adapt the game to suit your child's ability. When children are playing in a group, as many as possible should participate at the same time. All children get bored waiting in line, but children with mental retardation have even shorter attention spans. Group play often enhances these children's self-esteem as they experience being on equal footing with their peers. Likewise, group play, like team sports, helps children learn cooperation.

Focus on improvement, not on abilities. The less children are expected to do, the less they will do. Praise each milestone to encourage more success.

Children with mental retardation may have greater success in individual and dual sports than in team sports. Be consistent, and set clear rules for games and sportsmanship.

Teach by doing. Instead of explaining how to throw a ball, demonstrate, and then assist your child as he tries to do it—and do it, and do it. Be patient. Repetition often breeds competence. Teach one skill at a time. Once a child is comfortable with one technique, show him another.

Children with developmental disabilities develop many of the overuse injuries that afflict all athletes if they have poor training or neglect warm-up. They also are susceptible to heat stress if the enthusiasm for sport overshadows the ability to monitor fatigue and overheating. Be sure your child is closely supervised by a trained coach who can watch out for heat problems.

Half of moderately and severely retarded children have Down syndrome. About 15% of those children have an instability of the neck that results in serious injury if the neck is forced to bend. Although injuries of this type are uncommon from participation in sports, Special Olympics prohibits children with Down syndrome from participating in gymnastics, diving, the butterfly stroke in swimming, the high jump, the pentathlon, and soccer until they have been medically screened for atlantoaxial instability.

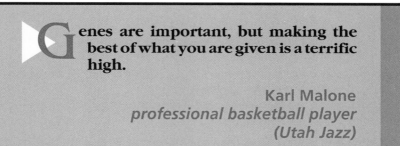

Genes are important, but making the best of what you are given is a terrific high.

Karl Malone
professional basketball player
(Utah Jazz)

To get your child with a developmental disability more involved in sports, contact the Special Olympics chapter nearest you. They should be listed in the telephone white pages, or contact the national headquarters at 1325 G Street NW, #500, Washington, DC 20005; phone 202-628-3630.

Working closely with health professionals will help you be sure your child, no matter what her current physical or mental condition, is getting the most out of her fitness program. As you can see, fitness and health go hand in hand. In the next chapter I'll help you assess the health of your family.

Organizations for Children With Special Needs

Achilles Track Club, 1 Times Sq., 10th Fl., New York, NY 10036; phone 212-354-0300

American Athletic Association for the Deaf, 3607 Washington Blvd. #4, Ogden, UT 84403-1737; phone 801-393-7916/(TDY) 807-393-8710

American Blind Skiing Foundation, 610 S. William St., Mt. Prospect, IL 60056; phone 708-255-1739

American Hearing Impaired Hockey Association, 1143 W. Lake St., Chicago, IL 60607; phone 312-226-5880

Alta Foundation, 3300 NE Expressway, #4L, Atlanta, GA 30341; phone 404-455-4141

Handicapped Scuba Association, 1104 El Prado, San Clemente, CA 92672; phone 714-498-6128 or 303-933-4864

National Amputee Golf Association, PO Box 5801, Coralville, IA 52241-5801; phone 800-633-6242

National Foundation of Wheelchair Tennis, 940 Calle Amanecer, #B, San Clemente, CA 92673; phone 714-361-6811

Disabled Sports USA, 451 Hungerford Dr., #100, Rockville, MD 20850; phone 301-217-0960

Wheelchair Sports USA, 3595 E. Fountain Blvd., Suite L1, Colorado Springs, CO 80910; phone 719-574-1150

National Wheelchair Basketball Association, University of Kentucky, 110 Seaton Building, Lexington, KY 40506; phone 606-276-2136

North American Riding for the Handicapped Association, PO Box 33150, Denver, CO 80233; phone 800-369-7433

Ski for Light, Inc., 1455 W. Lake St., Minneapolis, MN 55408; phone 612-827-3232

US Blind Golfers Association, 3094 Shamrock St. N., Tallahassee, FL 32308; phone 904-893-4511. Contact: Robert Andrews

Wilderness Inquiry, 1313 Fifth St. SE, Box 84, Minneapolis, MN 55414; phone 800-728-0719

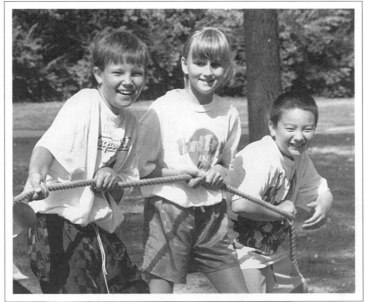

© Karen Maier

A Prescription for Family Fitness

Picture your child as an adult. In your mind's eye, do you see an energetic person with a zest for life that stems from respecting his or her body? By now you're well aware that fitness is an ongoing, lifetime process—there are no shortcuts. Many factors and behaviors affect your child's fitness. Your primary goal is to help your child develop healthy behaviors that will result in being fit now and maintaining that fitness throughout life, perhaps still running races at age 80!

Health is greatly influenced by how you live your life: what you do, and what you don't do. Healthy behaviors have great consequences, affecting moods, adding zest and energy, and often adding fruitful years to life. You can help your child now to be fit for the future by guiding him toward healthy choices. Let's review lifestyle choices you and your children can make to improve your health.

> Your health is really the most valuable asset of your life. Your fitness affects your self-image, and your view of yourself is more important than how others view you. You can't lie to yourself!
>
> Karl Malone
> *professional basketball player*
> *(Utah Jazz)*

Be Active and Eat Well

People who benefit most from physical activity are those who incorporate it into their daily lives. Just like brushing teeth or buckling a seat belt, an active lifestyle has to be a natural component of your child's day. Children who participate in physical education class, play on a community league team, and play actively with friends and family will reap the healthful benefits of exercise and develop interests that can stay with them well into their senior years.

What should you do? You've taken the first step by reading this book. Now try to implement this advice so that it becomes a natural extension of your family.

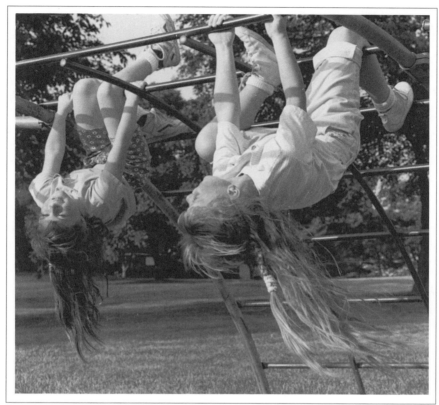

© Karen Maier

Each year researchers are finding more ways that diet relates to disease. I talked a lot in chapter 4 about how to help your child develop good eating habits and a healthy body composition. Helping your child learn to make healthy food choices is one of the greatest gifts you can give. Who wouldn't want to live a long life and never say *diet*. By helping your child acquire a taste for a healthy diet you can help them do just that.

Monitor Blood Pressure

Blood pressure gradually increases as people get older. Studies have shown that many adults with dangerously high blood pressure had childhood signs of hypertension. Lifestyle affects blood pressure. Both diet (too much fatty food as well as too many total calories) and activity (too little exercise) can push blood pressure too high. See Table 9.1 for healthy blood pressure levels for children of various ages.

Table 9.1 Healthy Blood Pressure in Children	
Age	Blood pressure
Under 6	Below 110/75
6 to 10	Below 120/80
11 to 14	Below 125/85
15 to 18	Below 135/90

Reprinted from Cooper (1991).

What do the numbers used to report blood pressure mean? The first, or systolic, number is the pressure of the blood against the vessel walls as the heart is pumping. The second, or diastolic, number is the pressure of the blood between beats when the heart is resting. An elevated reading in either number is cause for concern.

If your child has a high blood pressure reading, be sure the measurement was taken correctly. Was the blood pressure cuff snugly around the arm? An adult cuff often won't work correctly. Next, ask whether your child's developmental age is being taken into consideration. Chronological age isn't necessarily a true indicator of your child's development. Finally, be sure your child isn't suffering from "white coat" syndrome—becoming so nervous in the doctor's office that blood pressure rises, causing a falsely high reading. Try having your child's blood pressure taken in a less threatening environment.

If your child is confirmed as having high blood pressure, your doctor will recommend primarily a diet and exercise program. Salt intake is often restricted too. If this treatment doesn't work, especially if your family has a history of high blood pressure, drug therapy may be needed.

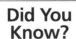

Did You Know?

Salt doesn't adversely affect most people's blood pressure. But it's too difficult and costly to test everyone, so doctors recommend that everyone restrict their salt intake.

Manage Stress

Childhood is often considered a time of carefree living and fun. But children often feel many of the same stresses their parents do. Family money problems, health concerns, and troubled relationships with family and friends can really stress a child. This stress, in turn, may lead to depression, low self-esteem, lowered immunities, and disease. Eating disorders are also linked to unhealthy levels of stress.

What is stressful to children? Here is a sampling of potential stressors:

- Accidents
- Arguments with friends or family
- Competition
- Death
- Disease
- Divorce
- Grades
- Ignorance

- Lack of money
- Latchkey living
- Loneliness
- Moving
- Peer pressure
- Problems with teachers
- Sports pressure

> When I had problems in school or with my parents, I played a set of tennis. The exercise made me feel strong mentally and emotionally, and I felt I could deal with my problems better.
>
> **Chris Evert**
> *professional tennis player*

Pay attention to your child to be sure stress isn't affecting her health. Symptoms of stress in children present themselves in a number of ways. You may notice your child is avoiding friends or withdrawing from you or other family members. She may seem unusually grumpy or complain frequently about headaches or stomachaches. In fact, overstressed kids are indeed sick a lot. Look for unexplained changes in eating habits, schoolwork, or athletic performance. Drug and alcohol use are often symptoms of stress, which can also develop into a rash of accidents or violent or rebellious behavior.

Don't belittle your child about his fears or concerns. Your child can develop unhealthy stress from real *or* imagined problems. Keep your lines of communication open so you can help your child cope. Many parents who exercise with their children find their workout sessions a perfect time to talk things out. A long walk or bike ride can let the mind wander; this relaxed state is ideal for bringing up troubling issues as well as gaining support for ideas.

Let your child know if you are worried about her and that you care deeply how she feels. Let her know that you've felt similar stress and that together you can work out any problem. If you can't help your child relax, talk to her teacher or doctor. Get help as soon as you feel you aren't making a difference. Most children are able to work out their problems with help, but some children have felt suicide to be the only answer.

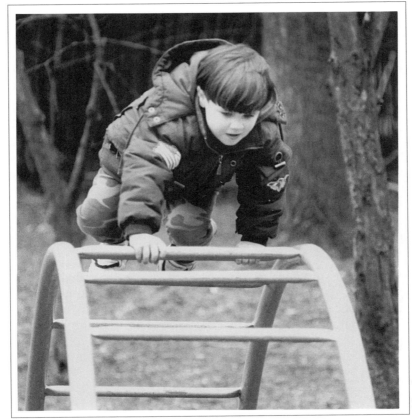

© Doug Brown

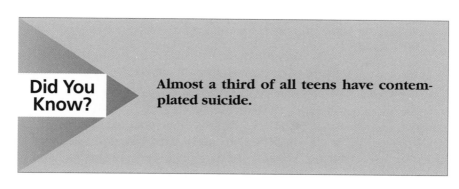

Did You Know? Almost a third of all teens have contemplated suicide.

Avoid Unhealthy Recreational Pursuits

I always hated when my parents began a discussion with "When I was your age . . ." Even so I must admit that when I was young it never crossed my mind to smoke cigarettes, drink alcohol, take illegal drugs, or become sexually active. Today these are all real options for children from every demographic background. Parents can combat these pressures head on by being good role models, having open and nonjudgmental discussions with their children, and keeping their eyes and ears open to possible problems.

Tobacco

The power of advertising and peer pressure is evident in the fact that people, mostly young women, are still taking up cigarette smoking. How can you help? Your first job is to set a good example. If you smoke, your child is twice as likely to smoke. So, first, stop smoking. Next, reinforce why smoking is bad. Don't simply focus on health problems caused by smoking—teens usually can't look past living until their mid-20s. Focus instead on the social ramifications of smoking: You smell bad, your teeth turn yellow, you get wrinkles early and squint too much. And don't forget that "kissing a smoker is like kissing an ashtray."

Many children try smoking. You may be unable to prevent this type of experimentation, but you can educate and motivate your child to prefer a different lifestyle. Few people who exercise also smoke. In fact, physical activity is recommended to smokers to help them quit smoking. If your child picks up the habit, work with your family doctor to develop a strategy to counter it.

> lowly incorporate healthy habits into your life. Look for ways to make activity part of your lifestyle. Run or walk or cycle with friends. Join a Y or other fitness center. Subscribe to magazines that explore health and fitness issues. Have faith in yourself, because you can and will become stronger and healthier if you try.
>
> Bill Rodgers
> *Olympic marathoner*

Alcohol, Drugs, and Sex

Too many parents aren't doing a good job teaching their children about alcohol and drug use and sex. Parents who are uncomfortable discussing these subjects with their children may ignore the issues until it's too late.

I've grouped these subjects because you should approach them with your child in the same way. They are all facts of life that your child needs your guidance with. They are also all schoolyard topics that your child will talk about with peers, regardless of your personal feelings. You need to arm your child with the facts, the self-esteem, and the courage to make healthy choices.

Begin discussions early, and never make them a big deal (unless abuse occurs). Preschoolers should be taught what they can and can't put into their mouths. Some things are good for you, other things aren't. They should learn that their bodies are private and precious. Children this age are aware that boys and girls have different sexual organs. To reduce inappropriate curious behavior, explain these differences openly using correct terminology and with a matter-of-fact tone.

Children in the early elementary years can be taught a little more. They should learn that medicine and drugs (including alcohol) affect the body. Used correctly, drugs make you feel better; used incorrectly, they make you sick. You should also acknowledge that some people do use medicine and drugs incorrectly. Your child may see a family member or friend tipsy at a social event. Acknowledge that the person is acting poorly, and explain that it is due to immoderate alcohol use.

During the elementary years your child can begin to learn about reproduction. Teach how all plants and animals reproduce. Explain the outcomes of sexual behavior: babies. And explain why sex should be limited to loving adults.

By junior high your child needs to understand thoroughly problems that can result from irresponsible drug use or irresponsible sex. Most parents think their children know less about these areas than they actually do. Children pick up information from television, their friends, and other family members—but these sources are not always accurate.

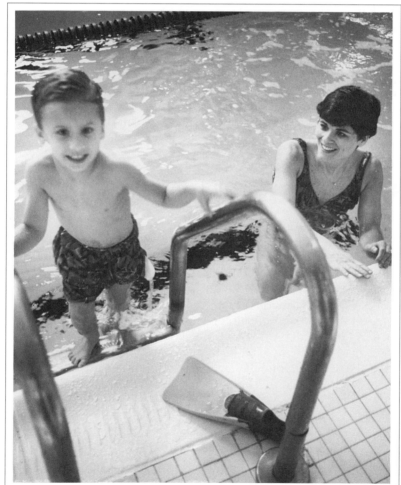

© Doug Brown

By always maintaining an open line of communication and talking matter-of-factly and honestly about sex and drug use, you will give your children the knowledge and self-esteem they need to weigh the pressures they feel in these areas and make healthful judgments.

Make Fitness an Everyday Venture

A fit lifestyle will be commonplace in the future. In our generation research has shown beyond the shadow of a doubt that a healthy lifestyle improves the quality and length of life. Doctors, teachers, and health educators are developing programs to make healthy choices like good eating and active living as taken for granted by future generations as brushing teeth is for baby boomers.

This book gives you the basics you need to develop a fit family. Now it's up to you. By preparing your child to take personal responsibility for health and fitness, you are giving one of the most precious gifts imaginable. By living healthfully and actively, your child will have the best chance possible to enjoy a long and happy life. What better gift can you give?

Complete Health Assessment

Health is not just the absence of disease, but a composite of many factors. In 1968, Richard Bohannon, MD, a former Surgeon General of the Air Force, founded the American Running and Fitness Association (formerly the National Jogging Association). AR&FA is a nonprofit educational association of recreational athletes and sports medicine professionals, helping Americans modify their behavior for better health. AR&FA developed the following health assessment test to help people identify what they do (or don't do) that affects their health. Have each family member take the test, then tabulate your results together. It will help your child to see that everyone has both strengths and weaknesses. Together, you can work to become healthier and happier.

American Running & Fitness Association (AR&FA) Health Assessment Test

Answer each question carefully, then total your points.

Exercise

1. How much time each week do you spend being active? This includes playing with friends or a team so that you get sweaty and your heart beats fast. It also includes walking briskly, running, cycling, swimming, aerobic dancing, rowing, cross-country skiing, and doing other aerobic activities (nonstop, vigorous exercise) as well as mowing the lawn, vacuuming, and other hard work. Sitting on the bench or watching other people work out doesn't count.

   a. 2-1/2 hours or more
   b. 1-1/2 to 2-1/2 hours
   c. 1 to 1-1/2 hours
   d. 30 minutes to 1 hour
   e. less than 30 minutes

2. Do you stretch your muscles?

   a. at least once a day   b. once a week
   c. sometimes   d. never

3. Do you warm up and cool down before you exercise?

   a. always   b. sometimes   c. never

4. Do you exercise in spite of pain?

   a. yes   b. no

5. Do you alternate hard and easy (or rest) days?

   a. yes   b. no

6. Do you strive for total-body fitness (endurance, strength, and flexibility) by doing a variety of activities?

   a. yes   b. no

Nutrition and diet

7. Do you eat a wide variety of foods (something from each of the four basic food groups: meat, fish, poultry, dried legumes, eggs, nuts; milk products; whole grain breads or cereals; fruits and vegetables)?

   a. every day
   b. at least three times a week
   c. once a week
   d. once in a while

8. Do you limit the amount of animal fat (butter, fatty meats) you eat?

   a. I avoid all animal fat.
   b. I don't each much animal fat (less than 10% of my calories come from these fats).
   c. I never really pay much attention to this; I don't try to avoid animal fat.
   d. I love fatty foods and eat them frequently.

9. Do you limit the amount of refined sugar (in candy, nondiet sodas, other sweets) you eat?

   a. I avoid refined sugar.
   b. I try to avoid it but occasionally have some.
   c. I never really pay much attention to these: I don't try to avoid refined sugar.
   d. I love refined-sugar products and eat them frequently.

10. Do you limit the amount of salt or salty foods in your diet?

    a. I avoid salt and salty foods.
    b. I try to avoid these but occasionally have some.
    c. I never really pay much attention to these; I don't try to avoid them.
    d. I love salt and salty foods and eat them frequently.

11. Do you eat a good breakfast (cereal, toast, fruit, and drink, for example)? Select what is closest to your typical pattern.

    a. I eat breakfast daily, with a light lunch and moderate dinner.
    b. I eat breakfast four days a week, with a light lunch and moderate dinner.
    c. I skip breakfast in favor of a light lunch and a heavy dinner.
    d. I skip breakfast and lunch and eat snacks during the day plus a heavy dinner.
    e. I snack all day and eat three heavy meals.
    f. I eat three heavy meals but do little snacking.
    g. I never really pay much attention to this.

12. Do you drink at least six to eight glasses of water a day?

    a. always   b. sometimes   c. never

Body composition

13. How much body fat do you have? Males should have 10% to 20% body fat, females 15% to 25%.

    a. My body fat is below the recommended range by more than two percentage points.
    b. My body fat is within +2 to –2 percentage points of recommendation.
    c. My body fat is within the recommended range.
    d. My body fat is 3 to 6 percentage points beyond the recommended range.
    e. My body fat is more than 6 percentage points beyond the recommended range.

14. Does your weight fluctuate much?

    a. I am under 18, my weight is slowly increasing. I maintain no more than the recommended body fat level.
    b. I am under 18, and my weight is slowly increasing. My body fat level is higher than recommended.
    c. My weight goes up and down throughout the year.
    d. I am over 18, and my weight has gone up and down over the years by more than 5 pounds.
    e. I am over 18, and my weight has stayed about the same for a number of years. I am within the recommended body fat levels.
    f. I am over 18, and my weight has stayed about the same for a number of years. My body fat is higher than recommended.

Smoking

15. Do you smoke?

    a. never
    b. I quit 2 or more years ago.
    c. I quit within the last year.
    d. I smoke 1 to 10 cigarettes or cigars a day (or a pipe).
    e. I smoke 11 to 20 cigarettes or cigars a day.
    f. I smoke more than 20 cigarettes or cigars a day.

Alcohol, drugs, and sex

16. Do you drink alcohol?

    a. never or almost never

    b. I am over 21 and drink 1 to 2 drinks a day

    d. I drink 3 to 4 drinks a day.

    e. I drink more than 4 drinks a day.

17. Do you get drunk?

    a. never

    b. 1 to 3 times a year

    c. 4 to 6 times a year

    d. more than 6 times a year

18. Do you use illegal drugs?

    a. never

    b. I am under 21 and use them infrequently.

    c. I am over 21 and use them infrequently.

    d. I use them once a month.

    e. I use them more than once a month.

19. Do you use prescription drugs?

    a. I rarely need or use them.

    b. I use them infrequently, as needed and prescribed by a physician.

    c. I don't follow the dosages or schedules prescribed.

    d. I regularly use non-prescription mood-altering drugs.

20. Do you understand and practice safe sex techniques?

    a. I am under age 12 and do not understand or practice safe sex techniques.

    b. I am over age 12 and understand safe sex techniques but am not sexually active.

    c. I am over age 12 and understand and practice safe sex techniques.

    d. I am over age 12 and do not understand safe sex techniques but am not sexually active.

    e. I am over age 12 and understand but do not practice safe sex techniques.

    f. I am over age 12 and do not understand and do not practice safe sex techniques.

Stress and relaxation

21. How much stress do you experience in your life?

a. very little
b. occasional mild tension
c. frequent mild tension
d. frequent moderate tension
e. frequent high tension

22. How secure and relaxed are you?

a. I'm always secure and relaxed.
b. I'm usually secure and relaxed.
c. I'm occasionally secure and relaxed.
d. I'm anxious or tense much of the time and have difficulty relaxing.

23. How much sleep do you get?

a. I am under 16 and get 6 to 7 hours a night.
b. I am 16 or older and get 6 to 7 hours at night.
c. I get 7 to 8 hours a night.
d. I am under 16 and get 8 to 12 hours a night.
e. I am 16 or older and get 8 to 9 hours a night.
f. I am under 16 and get more than 12 hours a night.
g. I am 16 or older and get more than 9 hours a night.
h. I get less than 6 hours a night.

Self-concept

24. How do you feel about yourself?

a. I feel good about myself and generally am confident about my future and my abilities.
b. I'm comfortable with myself and will probably do well in the future.
c. I'm usually comfortable with myself but have my ups and downs.
d. I'm not too happy with myself and seem to make too many mistakes.
e. I don't like myself and can't seem to do anything right.

25. How do you feel about your schoolwork or job? (Homemakers are professionals too!)

    a. It's challenging and I enjoy it.

    b. It's sometimes challenging and I'm usually content with it.

    c. It's what I have to do.

    d. I don't like my schoolwork or job.

    e. I hate my schoolwork or job.

26. Have any of the following happened to you within the last year? (Circle all that apply.)

    a. death of a family member, friend, or close relative

    b. change of residence

    c. school or career change

    d. parents' or personal divorce or separation

Medical care

27. How often do you visit a doctor for a checkup?

    a. I am under 18 and go once a year.

    b. I am under 18 and go once every 2 or 3 years.

    c. I am over 18 and go once every 2 or 3 years.

    d. I go once every 4 years or so.

    e. I rarely or never go.

28. If you have reached puberty, do you do breast or testicular self-exams?

    a. monthly   b. occasionally

    c. never   d. I have not reached puberty.

29. Is your cholesterol level in the healthy range?

    a. yes   b. no   c. I don't know my level.

30. Is your blood pressure level in the healthy range?

    a. yes   b. no   c. I don't know my level.

✓Scoring

1. a. 18   b. 17   c. 16   d. 8   e. 0
2. a. 3   b. 2   c. 1   d. 0
3. a. 1   b. 0   c. −2
4. a. −5   b. 0
5. a. 0   b. −1
6. a. 3   b. 0
7. a. 10   b. 7   c. −5   d. −10
8. a. 7   b. 10   c. 0   d. −5
9. a. 2   b. 1   c. 0   d. −1
10. a. 2   b. 1   c. 0   d. −1
11. a. 3   b. 1   c. −1   d. −2   e. −10   f. −4   g. −4
12. a. 3   b. 1   c. −1
13. a. −2   b. 5   c. 10   d. −5   e. −10
14. a. 2   b. −1   c. −3   d. −3   e. 2
15. a. 4   b. 3   c. 2   d. −4   e. −6   f. −10
16. a. 0   b. 0   c. −5   d. −2   e. −5
17. a. 2   b. −1   c. −3   d. −5
18. a. 2   b. −1   c. −1   d. −5   e. −7   f. −7
19. a. 2   b. 0   c. −3   d. −7
20. a. 0   b. 0   c. 0   d. −1   e. −3   f. −5
21. a. 2   b. 0   c. −1   d. −2   e. −4
22. a. 2   b. 0   c. −1   d. −3
23. a. −1   b. 0   c. 1   d. 1   e. 0   f. −1   g. −1   h. −3
24. a. 2   b. 1   c. 0   d. −1   e. −3
25. a. 2   b. 1   c. 0   d. −1   e. −3
26. a. −5   b. −2   c. −1   d. −3
27. a. 2   b. −2   c. 2   d. −3   e. −10
28. a. 0   b. −1   c. −3   d. 0
29. a. 4   b. −2   c. −2
30. a. 4   b. −2   c. −2

✓Results

Over 87—Great job! Keep up the good work.

70 to 87—Good job! You are making a positive impact on your health.

50 to 69—Not bad, but you can do better. By making a stronger commitment to a healthy lifestyle you will improve your mental and physical health.

Under 69—Not good—but at least you are reading this book. Begin making changes now and you can greatly improve your health and fitness.

Recommended Reading

The Aerobics Program for Total Well-Being by Ken Cooper, 1982, New York: M. Evans and Company.

ACSM Fitness Book by the American College of Sports Medicine, 1992, Champaign, IL: Human Kinetics.

Anybody's Guide to Total Fitness by Len Kravits, 1986, Dubuque, IA: Kendal Hunt.

Coaching Young Athletes by Rainer Martens, Robert Christina, John Harvey, Jr., and Brian Sharkey, 1981, Champaign, IL: Human Kinetics.

Complete Guide to Youth Fitness Testing by Margaret Safrit, 1995, Champaign, IL: Human Kinetics.

Exercise and Children's Health by Thomas Rowland, 1990, Champaign, IL: Human Kinetics.

Kid Fitness by Ken Cooper, 1991, New York: Bantam Books.

Nancy Clark's Sports Nutrition Guidebook by Nancy Clark, 1990, Champaign, IL: Human Kinetics.

The New Fit or Fat by Covert Bailey, 1991, Boston: Houghton Mifflin.

Nutrition, Weight Control, and Exercise by Frank Katch and William McKardle, 1988, Boston: Houghton Mifflin.

Parents Guide to Feeling Good by Charles Kuntzleman, 1982, Spring Arbor, MI: Feeling Good.

Power Foods by Liz Applegate, 1991, Emmaus, PA: Rodale Press.

Sensible Fitness by Jack Wilmore, 1986, Champaign, IL: Human Kinetics.

Sport First Aid by Melinda Flegel, 1992, Champaign, IL: Human Kinetics.

Sport Parent by American Sport Education Program, 1995, Champaign, IL: Human Kinetics.

Sport Selection by Robert Arnot and Charles Gains, 1984, New York: Viking Press.

Sport Stretch by Michael Alter, 1990, Champaign, IL: Human Kinetics.

SportsTalent by Robert Arnot and Charles Gaines, 1984, New York: Viking Press.

The Stanford Health and Exercise Handbook by Stanford Alumni Association, 1987, Champaign, IL: Human Kinetics.

Strength Training for Young Athletes by William Kraemer and Steven Fleck, 1993, Champaign, IL: Human Kinetics.

The Well Family Book by Charles Kuntzleman, 1985, San Bernardino, CA: Here's Life.

Index

About the Author

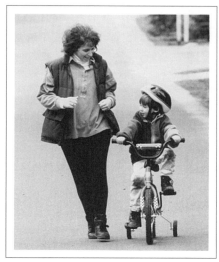

© Doug Brown

Susan Kalish is the executive Director of the American Running and Fitness Association (AR&FA), a national nonprofit educational association of recreational athletes, and also is the executive director of the American Medical Athletic Association, a national nonprofit educational association of medical professionals who have a personal interest in physical fitness. Together these groups develop educational and motivational programs to encourage more Americans to become fit.

Susan has been editor-in-chief of *Running & FitNews*—a monthly newsletter that reports on sports medicine, nutrition, and health research— since 1983. She has developed a number of national programs to encourage people to exercise and help them maintain their exercise programs, including Exercise Across America, Share the Road, AR&FA Sportsmedicine Referral Network, AR&FA Running Shoe Database, and AR&FA Exercise Trails Network. In addition, she has written numerous articles on exercise, training, and diet for such publications as *Encyclopedia Britannica*, *Running Times*, *Women's Sports & Fitness*, and the *Washington Business Journal*. She is also the author of *The New AR&FA MultiSport Log Book*.

Susan is on the Board of Advisors of the Rails to Trails Conservancy and the American Volksmarch Association. She also serves on the editorial board for *Shape* magazine, the steering committee for Healthy People 2000 Physical Activity Components, and the ad hoc committee for organizing the Marine Corps Marathon. Susan lives in Fairfax, VA, with her husband, John McMahon, and her two children, Matthew and Alexa.

More HK books for parents and their children

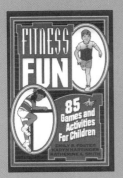

Fitness Fun

Emily R. Foster, MAT, Karyn Hartinger, MS, and Katherine A. Smith, MS

1992 • Paper • 112 pp • Item BFOS0384
ISBN 0-87322-384-5 • $12.95 ($17.95 Canadian)

Contains 85 field-tested games and activities that will help maximize fitness in children.

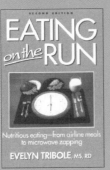

Eating on the Run

(Second Edition)
Evelyn Tribole, MS, RD

Foreword by Barbara Harris, editor of *Shape* magazine

1992 • Paper • 256 pp • Item PTRI0452
ISBN 0-88011-452-5 • $14.95 ($21.95 Canadian)

Provides the nutrition information necessary for making healthy eating choices, even when time is limited.

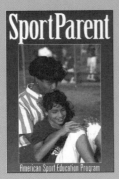

SportParent

American Sport Education Program

1994 • Paper • 96 pp • Item ACEP0452
ISBN 0-87322-696-8 • $8.95 ($11.95 Canadian)

Shows parents how they can become active partners with coaches to provide children with beneficial, enjoyable, and safe sport experiences.

To place your order, U.S. customers call **TOLL-FREE 1 800 747-4457**.
Customers outside the U.S. place your order using the appropriate telephone number/address shown in the front of this book.

Prices subject to change.

 Human Kinetics
The Premier Publisher for Sports & Fitness

2335

DATE DUE

DE 06			
OC 13 09			

Demco, Inc. 38-293

Executive   ssociation

Human Kinetics

and Johnnie Angel,
and patience.

Library of Congress Cataloging-in-Publication Data

Kalish, Susan, 1958–
    Your child's fitness: practical advice for parents / Susan
    Kalish.
       p. cm.
    Includes bibliographical references and index.
    ISBN 0-87322-540-6
    1. Physical fitness for children.   I. Title.
   GV443.K26   1995
   361.7'042--dc20   95-8976
                                           CIP

ISBN: 0-87322-540-6

Developmental Editors: Anne Mischakoff Heiles, Nanette Smith; **Assistant Editors:** Kirby Mittelmeier, Henry Woolsey, and Ann Greenseth; **Editorial Assistant:** Alecia Mapes Walk; **Copyeditor:** Molly Bentsen; **Proofreader:** Karen Bojda; **Indexer:** Theresa J. Schafer; **Typesetter:** Francine Hamerski; **Text Designer:** Robert Reuther; **Layout Artists:** Francine Hamerski and Robert Reuther; **Cover Designer:** Jack Davis; **Photographer (cover):** Photo Network/Michael Philip Manheim; **Photographers (interior):** Doug Brown, Bruce Barthel, and Karen Maier; **Illustrator:** Keith Blomberg; **Printer:** United Graphics

Human Kinetics books are available at special discounts for bulk purchase. Special editions or book excerpts can also be created to specification. For details, contact the Special Sales Manager at Human Kinetics.

Printed in the United States of America   10 9 8 7 6 5 4 3 2 1

Human Kinetics
P.O. Box 5076, Champaign, IL 61825-5076
1-800-747-4457

Canada: Human Kinetics, Box 24040, Windsor, ON N8Y 4Y9
1-800-465-7301 (in Canada only)

Europe: Human Kinetics, P.O. Box IW14, Leeds LS16 6TR, United Kingdom
(44) 1132 781708

Australia: Human Kinetics, 2 Ingrid Street, Clapham 5062, South Australia
(08) 371 3755

New Zealand: Human Kinetics, P.O. Box 105-231, Auckland 1
(09) 523 3462